FUNDAMENTAL MAXIMS OF AYURVEDA

Adoration to Gaṇeśa. Adoration to Saraswati

Govinda Vadanāmbhoja Taruṇāruṇa Sarathiḥ

Cakāsta Hṛdaye Śaśvād Gururme Guṇinām Varaḥ

Let Govinda, charioteer, whose face is blossoming red lotus, my Guru (teacher) who is the treasure of all righteousness, may reside in my heart for ever.

Though the sun himself is luminous, he is charioteered by a teacher who is more luminous with all righteousness.

My teacher is Govinda who had a great Guru. Let Him also reside in my heart for ever.

NAMĀMI DHANAVANTARIM ADIVEVAM
SURĀSURAIH VANDITA PĀDA PADAM
LOKE JARÄ RUGBAYA MRTYU NĀŚAM
DHĀTĀRAMĪSĀM VIVIDHAUSADHĪNĀM

I salute Lord DHANVANTARI, the foremost God, Gods as well as devils (others) bow down at His lotus-like feet. He holds various medicines that control old age, cure disease, prohibit phobias and death.

Hari Shri Gaṇapataye Namah Avighnamastu
Om Namo Nārāyaṇāya

FUNDAMENTAL MAXIMS OF AYURVEDA

(Prepared for the common people)

S.V. Govindan

ABHINAV PUBLICATIONS

abhinav publications
New Delhi

First published in India 2003

Publishers
Shakti Malik
ABHINAV PUBLICATIONS
E-37, Hauz Khas
New Delhi - 110 016 (INDIA)
Phones: 6566387, 6562784, 6524658
Fax: 91-11-6857009
e-mail: shakti@nde.vsnl.net.in
website: www.abhinavexports.com

ISBN 81-7017-417-1

Lasertypeset by
S.R. Enterprises
Lajpat Nagar-IV
New Delhi-110024

Printed at
D.K. Fine Art Press Pvt. Ltd.
Ashok Vihar
Delhi

CONTENTS

Foreword 7

Introduction 9

Chapters

1 **Ayurveda** *11*
2 **Tridosa (Three Humours) Theory** *19*
3 **Importance of Matters** *47*
4 **Maternity and Pediatrics** *69*
5 **Prediction by Observing the Symptoms** *87*
6 **Diagnosis** *95*
7 **About the Body** *109*
8 **Pancakarma in a Nutshell** *121*
9 **Some Diseases and their Treatment** *135*

Index *151*

FOREWORD

Shri S.V. Govindan known as "Govindanji" is more a saint than a common man. "Simple life and high thinking" is being practised throughout his life successfully and so a man of sanctity. He is an acclaimed expert in Yoga and Massage techniques.

When I came to know about his effort on a book about Ayurvedic principles, I, naturally, was very eager to go through it. Though this book is intended for laymen according to the author, but on going through it, I feel that it is useful even for a professional.

A book can be said to be useful if we get a lot of information or can gain a compilation of scattered bits of datas. In this respect this book is very beneficial. The vastness of the subject and the simple way of approach may cause some problem to laymen to move ahead smoothly in the first chapter but as we advance things change and the matter turns to be quite absorbing.

When I went through it for the first time I thought to tell him to strike off the list of books regarding each branch of Ayurveda. But on a second thought I dropped this idea, because it will be useful for a professional in many ways.

The chapters are arranged in a unique order as to make the progression savoury. The signs of good and bad messengers and symptoms of nearing death are not commonly dealt with in ayurvedic books for common people. But proper significance is given to that subject in this book, which is very advantageous.

Selection of datas, mode of compilation and the nature of language followed in this book are admirable. These features make the book worthwhile for laymen as well as professionals.

Before concluding I would like to appreciate and admire the effort Govindanji has made in releasing such a work and certainly he has carved out for himself an honourable place in the succession of ayurvedic writers by the release of this book.

Changanacherry
9.4.2002

Dr. M.C. Vijayachandra Das
Sree Sankara Hospital,
Changanacherry, Kerala

INTRODUCTION

When I was first invited to Germany in 1986, my friend Mr. Peter Ruhe arranged a meeting in Berlin, in which I had to speak on Ayurveda. I requested him to change the subject as I didn't know anything about Ayurveda except something about Ayurvedic Massage. He replied that it would not be possible as more than twenty-five doctors had already been informed by phone that they would attend the conference. I could not find any book on Ayurveda in English or in Hindi to refer to. Really I prayed the Almighty to help me. I prepared my talk in writing covering 7-8 pages which was enough for 40-45 minutes. I touched vata, pitta, kapha, the tridosa, some of the special treatments of Kerala like Navarakkizhi, Pizhichil and just mentioned the purification process of Pancakarma without any explanation. My talk was translated sentence by sentence into German language. So it took about 90 minutes altogether. After my speech, a German lady doctor who had read about Ayurveda also spoke for about 30 minutes. So the audience were satisfied.

During my journey I had seen several Ayurvedic books in German, Italian and French. I had also seen the costly books of Dr. Deepak Chopra and Dr. Vasant Lad on Ayurveda, and the audience began to appreciate my talks. I thought it would be better for the common people to understand Ayurveda if I could publish it.

I should mention some of the important authors and works that I had referred to for this work. They are: Agrivesa, Atreya, Bhadra Saunaka, Bhela, Bhoja, Candra Nandana, Caraka, Cikitsa Kalika, Cikitsa Sara Sangraha, Cintamaṇi, Dalhana, Garga, Gopura, Hariscandra, Harita, Jejjata, Kasyapa, Krsnatreya, Ksarapani, Kharanada, Narapati Carya, Nagarjuna, Padma, Prayoga Parijata, Ratnakara, Rasa Ratnakara, Rasa Sara, Rasa Siddhanta, Rasarnava, Rudra Kautuka, Rudra Tantra, Raudramsa, Sarrigadhara, Sivagama, Sivamekhala, Saunaka, Siddha Sara, Susruta, Vasistha, Vagbhata, Vacaspati, Videha, Viveka Martanda, Visvamitra, Vīrabhadra, Vaikhanasa, Vaidyalankara, Vaisvanara, Yoga Pradipa, Yoga Ratnavali, Yoga Sastra etc. I am grateful to all of them.

When I prepared the copy for publication, I contacted Mr. Shakti Malik, Abhinav Publications, New Delhi, who had published my first book "Ayurvedic Massage", and he agreed to publish it. So I am thankful to him.

Dr. R. Sreekumar, one of my grand nephews, helped me a lot for the computer work.

I sincerely hope that this book will enlighten the readers who are interested in Ayurveda and leaving the antibiotic medicines come forward for the Ayurvedic treatment which is really a holistic treatment.

Lokah Samastah Sukhino Bhavantu.

Bangalore
2nd Oct., 2001

S.V. Govindan
Brahma Vidya Mandir
Paunar (WARDHA)
INDIA
Tel: 0091 7152 43518

Chapter 1

AYURVEDA

AIMS AND OBJECTS

The body is the vehicle to achieve four-fold objects of human life, religious virtue, wealth and objects of senses, satisfaction of worldly desires and salvation. The bodies are controlled by Prana (elan vital). Diseases bring about morbidity in elan vital. To prevent and cure the diseases by treatment great scholars have composed texts on Ayurveda.

DEFINITION OF AYURVEDA

The science by which scholars could ascertain the factors that are useful and harmful for life and causative factors as well as the treatment of diseases is called Ayurveda.

There are eight branches of Ayurveda:

Surgery: Treatment of wounds caused by the injury to the body through weapons is called Salya (Surgery) for which blunt instruments, alkalies, cauterisation, sharp edged instruments, drugs and wholesome diet are used. The painful ailments caused by the vitiated waste products are also called surgery.

Probes (Salakya) or treatment of diseases of head and neck: The treatment of diseases of head and neck is generally done by probes.

Treatment of poisoning (Agada Tantra): Treatment of various types of poisons of vegetable and mineral origin, animal origin, prepared by combination of different drugs is called treatment of poisoning (Agada).

Maternity and Pediatrics (Kumara Bharana): The management of pregnancy and child after delivery, selection of wet-nerve, defect in breast milk and their corrections, signs and symptoms of afflictions by evil planets and their treatment and treatment of diseases during ailments of women during delivery is called treatment of maternity and pediatrics..

Treatment of internal diseases (Kaya cikitsa): Digestive fire of living beings is called kaya. Hence the treatment of diseases caused by suppression or irregularities of the digestive fire is called treatment of intestinal diseases. The prevention and treatment of diseases which pervade the entire body like fever, insanity, obstinate urinary disorders including diabetes, gout, bleeding from different parts of the body, obstinate skin diseases and leprosy, diarrhea, oedema, constipation, anaemia, anoreia, adiposity, piles, colic pain, obstinate abdominal diseases and ascites and genital organs is called kaya cikitsa or treatment of internal diseases.

Treatment of afflictions by evil spirits (Bhuta Kriya): Performance of propitious rituals, sacrifice rituals, oblation to the fire, charity to propitiate gods, demons, planets, dead ancestors etc., when they afflict the body is called treatment of afflictions by evil spirits. The treatment in the form of tying by ropes, controlling measures, biting, inhalation therapy, collyrium and fumigation is called Bhuta cikitsa.

Science of aphrodisiacs (Vajikarana): Factors which are responsible for increase in quantity, purification, accumulation, ejaculation and nourishment of semen which has become less in quantity, vitiated, diminished and dried are called aphrodisiacs.

Science of rejuvenation (Rasayana): The therapy that is administered for producing sturdiness of the body, the semen and teeth, which prevents wrinkles in the skin, graying of hair and baldness, and which promotes intellect as well as longevity is called science of rejuvenation (Rasayana).

The nourishment of the channels of circulation of plasma, hemoglobin fraction of the blood etc. is called rejuvenation.

There are several texts of great scholars on each branch in the name of samhitas, tantras etc. Some of the texts on each branch are:

Internal medicine (Kaya Cikitsa): Caraka Samhita, Ashtanga Samhita, Ashtanga Hrdaya, Aswini Kumara Samhita etc.

General Surgery (Salya): Dhanvantari Samhita, Susruta Samhita, Bhoja Tantra, Kapila Tantra etc.

Treatment for diseases of Head and Neck (Salakya): Videha Tantra, Saunaka Tantra, Karala Tantra etc.

Maternity and Pediatrics (Kumara Bharana): Parvataka Tantra, Bauddhaka Tantra, Kumara Tantra etc.

Poisoning (Toxicology) (Agada Tantra): Kasyapa Samhita, Sanaka Samhita, Garuda Samhita etc.

Science of aphrodisiacs (Vajikarana): Kucumana Tantra

Science of Rejuvenation (Rasayana)

Treatment of afflictions by evil spirits (Bhuta Kriya): Caraka and Susruta have dealt with these branches also in their samhitas. In respect of these branches names of works are not available.

The four limbs responsible for the accomplishment of treatment are: the physician, the patient, the drugs and medicines, and attendants and nurses.

The physician should have the following attributes:

Knowledge of the meanings and essence of medical texts

Experience of observations of the administration of therapeutics

Experience of self-administration of therapeutics

Very swift hand in administration of therapeutics

Purity

Bravery

Possession of all implements and drugs

Presence of mind

Intelligence

Enterprising nature

Sincerity in efforts

Observance of the path of truth and virtue

Qualities of nurse: Attachment, purity, more expertise and intelligence.

Qualities of patient: Possession of wealth, obedience to the physician, ability to express the complaints, strong will-power, suitable body for different treatments prescribed for the disease, age, sex and self-control.

Curability of disease depends upon eleven characteristic features:

Non-involvement of marma (vital spots) in the manifestation of diseases

Diseases which are caused by less numbers of etiological factors

Diseases having less of premonitory signs and symptoms

Diseases which have less of manifested signs and symptoms

Absence of complication

Dissimilarity among the afflicted tissue elements, locality, nature of season and physical constitution of the patient

Availability of excellence of physician, drugs, nurse and the patient

Favourable disposition of the planets

Involvement of only one channel in the pathogenesis of the disease

Disease which has occurred recently

Improvement of only one humour in the manifestation of disease

Fever is curable when the nature of humours and the season are similar. Obstinate urinary disorder including diabetes is curable if the humours are similar in nature to that of afflicted tissue elements. Rakta Gulma (chronic enlargement of spleen) is curable in its chronic stage.

The genuine physicians, who are accomplished in the administration of therapy, insight and knowledge of therapeutics, who are endowed with infallible success, and who give happiness to the patients are the saviours of life.

Curable diseases of patients engaged in penance or vedic rituals, who hide their diseases, young children and who constantly remain with a king or VIPs do not get cured easily. So they should be treated very carefully.

Three categories of physical and psychic diseases are:

as a result of past actions
due to aggravation of humours
both past actions and aggravation of humours

Diseases that transmigrate from one life to other are:

Obstinate skin diseases, leprosy
Obstinate urinary diseases, diabetes
Obstinate abdominal diseases, acidity
Leucoderma
Obstinate fever
Insanity
Fistula in ano
Other diseases like tuberculosis

These diseases transmigrate though they are suppressed. The transmigration does not take place if the body is cleaned well.

Diseases are classified into various categories:

Depending on the aggravation of humours of wind, bile and mucus

Depending on the location—body and mind

Depending on the amenability to treatment—curable, palliable and incurable

Curables are:

easily curable

curable with difficulty

Incurables are:

palliable

absolutely incurable

Characteristic features of curable diseases: (a) aggravation of humour, (b) free from complication, (c) strong power of digestion and metabolism, (d) strong will-power of self-confidence, (e) wealthy, (f) proper treatment administered, and (g) non-chronic diseases.

Three types of examination: (a) spiritual testimony including words and sages, (b) direct observation and (c) inference including reasoning.

Eyes, ears, tongue, nose, skin are examined and also asking questions.

Susruta's classification of diseases: (a) inherited diseases, (b) congenital diseases, (c) aggravation of humours, (d) vagaries of time and seasonal changes, (e) injuries, (f) providential factors, and (g) natural diseases.

Categories of diseases: (a) Adhyatmika (arising out of one's own self), (b) Adhibhautika (arising out of external objects), and (c) Adhidaivika (arising out of providential causes.

Diseases arising out of one's own self are: (a) hereditary—as a result of vitiation of the sperm and ovum of the parents, leprosy, piles and similar diseases from mother or from father, (b) congenital— resulting from improper diet and regimen of the mother during the period of gestation, for example, blindness, immobility of limbs, dumbness, impotency, stammering or lulling speech, dwarfism etc., vitiation of plasma of the mother and improper management of the mother during bicardiac stage of pregnancy, (c) as a result of wrong diet and regimen of the individual, diseases of stomach and upper portion of the intestine, diseases of large intestine.

Arising out of external objects: diseases by affliction of external objects, extraneous, by wild animals and by weapons.

Arising out of providential causes: (a) as a result of rainy, cold or hot seasons, out of wind, sun ray, vagaries of seasons, and normal seasons, (b) diseases due to the displeasure of gods: (i) contagious, (ii) evil tantric rites, (iii) lightning and fire, (iv) evil spirit (contagious or epidemic diseases), and (v) accidental.

Natural diseases: hunger, thirst, old age, sleep, ego, passion etc.

Chapter 2

TRIDOSA (THREE HUMOURS) THEORY

Science is a collection of successful recipes in methodological manner and all sciences analyze the material world from different viewpoints and angles. In Indian science, a philosophical approach can be seen very clearly; the philosophical background is common for arts, sciences and technology.

Ayurveda approaches the human body only as a modified reflection of external environment. So reflection of sun, moon and wind etc., the external environment can be seen in human body. Wind represents the transporting and regulating force, sun represents energy source and moon represents material source. These three concepts are respectively represented by Vata (wind), Pitta (bile) and Kapha (mucus) in living body and this gross approach is more philosophical in its nature. In fact they are three windows through which we can observe, analyze and find solutions to almost all human nature and illness.

For proper functioning of any mechanical or biological system three factors are necessary, a structural formation, energy conversion system and regulatory system; in human body these factors are represented by Kapha (mucus), Pitta (bile) and Vata (wind) respectively. A balanced state of these factors leads to perfect health, and imbalance stage of any one of these is called Dosa (humour) and leads to illness. In the working of any mechanical biological system there must be three factors: (a) structural formation, (b) energy conversion, and (c) regulatory system.

A genuine physician knows accumulation, aggravation, overflowing, lodgement in a particular place, manifestation, and classification or dissolution of these humours. In normal condition they sustain the body and in abnormal condition they destroy it. Though these humours pervade all over the body, mucus is located above cardiac region, bile is located between cardiac and umbilical region, and wind is located below umbilical region. Wind, bile, and mucus get aggravated during the end, middle, and beginning of the daytime, respectively. The same circle continues during night and during digestion also. Any kind of substance is known only through its properties. The great five elements contain a group properties. The ancient sages made a logical grouping of these properties as Vata, Pitta and Kapha which are biological neglections of satwa, raja and tama.

All visible and invisible happenings of the universe are under the influence of Cosmic impulse (Prana). There are five kinds of Prana and each has its region to control:

Prana: Its region is between larynx and the base of the heart. It governs the verbal mechanism, vocal apparatus, movements of gullet, respiratory system and the corresponding muscles. Its normal function is to receive all incoming impulses and to control unconsciously the activity of the sympathetic fibres. It is situated in medulla oblongata and governs the respiratory and circulatory functions. It rules the region between mouth and heart.

Apana: It dwells below the navel and rules the actions of kidney, the colon, the rectum, the bladder and the genital. These functions are governed by impulses from the lumbar portion. Normally it sends outgoing impulses to the excretory and ejaculatory mechanisms. These impulses cause relaxation of the sphincters of the anus and bladder as well as contraction of the muscular portion above them. These actions are necessary for the expulsion.

Samana: Its location is in the region between the heart and the navel, and rules the machinery of metabolism for the maintenance of life, the secretion of the stomach, the liver, the pancreas and the intestine, circulation of blood in the heart and the blood vessels. It is controlled by splanchnic nerves arising out of the ganglia in the thorax region. It inhibits the excessive activity of the digestive tract.

Udana: As it rules the region above the larynx, it keeps us on the alert regarding our special senses. All automatic functions of anatomical sections are under control of the cephalic division. As the thalamus is the highest reflex centre in the brain and all impressions ascend to it, it is called Udana. By conscious control over it all outgoing and incoming sensations can be suppressed. The suppression is necessary to prevent the distraction of the mind.

Vyana: It pervades the whole body and governs the movements of the body, contraction and relaxation of the muscles (voluntary and involuntary) and the joints etc. It is responsible for the erect posture of the body, reflex action through the spinal cord and through the stimulation of the autonomic ganglia. Its function is to keep the body in stationary condition which is due to balancing of action of the antogonic muscles through the unconscious reflexes that are generated along the spinal cord.

Qualities of water: Life giving, satiating, comforting to the heart and mind, refreshing, stimulating the intellect, unclear taste, cold in potency, light and like nectar of life.

Qualities of cold water: Relieves alcoholic intoxication, fainting, vomiting, debility, exhaustion, giddiness, thirst, burning sensation, aggravation of Pitta (bile), blood and toxins.

Qualities of hot water: Stimulates hunger, good for throat, hot in potency, diuretic for hiccup, distended abdomen, wind and mucus disorders, recent fever, cough, ama, flowing nose, dyspnoea and pain in flanks.

Qualities of coconut water: Unctuous, sweet, aphrodisiac, cold in potency, increases Agni (digestive fire) and it is diuretic.

Qualities of milk: Sweet in taste and Vipaka, unctuous, invigorating (good for ojas), nourishes dhatus, reduces wind and bile, it is aphrodisiac. Increases mucus, heavy and cold in potency.

Qualities of cow's milk: Promotes long life, rejuvenator, and good for emaciated ones after injury. Increases intelligence and strength as breast milk. Helps in easy movements of bowels, cures exhaustion, dizziness, toxicity, dyspnoea, relieves thirst and hunger, long-standing fever, diarrhea and bleeding diseases.

Qualities of buffalo's milk: More heavy, cold, unctuous; hence good for those who have excessive digestive fire and reduces sleep.

Qualities of goat's milk: More light, cures emaciating diseases, fever, dyspnoea, bleeding disease and diarrhea.

Qualities of camel milk: Slightly non-unctuous, hot in potency, salty, increases hunger, easily digestible, helps to increase wind and mucus, ascites, worms and hemorrhoids.

Qualities of mother's milk: Relieves aggravation of wind, bile and mucus, and blood. Cures traumatic wounds and eye-diseases.

Qualities of curd (yoghurt): Sour taste and at the end of digestion (Vipaka) heavy, hot in potency, reduces wind, increases Medha, semen, strength, mucus, bile, blood and digestive fire and inflammations. Improves tastes, intermittent fever, chronic rheumatics, dysuria. Don't use at night, and don't heat it in spring and autumn.

Qualities of buttermilk: Light, astringent and sour. Increases digestive fire, reduces mucus and wind. Cures oedema, ascites, hemorrhoids, grahini, dysuria, loss of appetite, enlargement of spleen and complication of excess consumption of clarified butter.

Qualities of butter: Aphrodisiac and cold in potency. Improves complexion, strength, and digestion. Cures paralysis and cough.

Qualities of honey: Good for eyes, breaks up hard masses. Relieves thirst, mucus, poison, hiccup, bleeding, diabetes, skin diseases, worm, vomiting, dyspnoea, cough, diarrhea. Heals wounds, increases wind.

Sweet and slightly astringent in taste. Don't use while hot, suffering from great heat, during hot season and also with hot food.

Qualities of oils

1. **Sesame oil:** Little bitter, flowing, subtle, hot, not good for eyes. Does not increase mucus; sesame (gingili) makes obese lean. Destroys worm. With appropriate processing with medicines it cures diseases.
2. **Castor oil:** Bitter, pungent, and sweet taste, laxative, heavy. Cures enlargement of abdomen, diseases of wind and mucus, intermittent fever, pain and swelling of waist, genitals, abdomen and back. It is capable of penetrating deep; hot in potency and bad in smell.
3. **Mustard oil:** Pungent, hot in potency. Reduces mucus, semen, tissue elements and wind. It improves digestive fire, produces bleeding diseases and other skin diseases.
4. **Margosa oil (Neem oil):** Slightly hot, bitter; destroys worm and microbes. Cures leprosy and other skin diseases, and reduces mucus.

Qualities of fermented rice water (water after washing rice for cooking): Sara, pungent; increases bile and hunger; cures pain in urinary bladder, and reduces wind and mucus.

Qualities of Soyas

1. **Green soya:** Best among legumes; mildly increases wind. Astringent in taste, cold in potency, easy to digest. Reduces mucus and bile. Suitable for external use also during bath.

2. **Black soya:** Unctuous, heavy, sara, hot in potency, sweet, increases strength, mucus and bile, and eliminates semen greatly.

Food stuffs: favourable and avoidable

Vata (Wind)

Favourable	Avoidable
Rice, wheat, green soya, black soya, sesame, oats	Chick-pea, yellow soya, brown soya, barley
Nutmeg, asafoetida, dried ginger, pepper, ajwain, garlic, saffron, cumin, clove and fenugreek	Coriander leaves, turmeric and coriander seed
Snake gourd, ash gourd, asparagus, brinjal, onion, carrot, beetroot, tomato, green chilly, gooseberry, and cucumber	Tender mango, beans, sprouts, broccoli, cauliflower, ladies finger, bitter gourd, tapioca, zucchini, potato, peas, cabbage, celery and leaf-vegetables
Papaya, apricot, orange, avocado, banana, cherries, lemon, coconut, pomegranate, figs, pineapple, plums and dates	Jamboline, apple, unripe jackfruit, dried fruits, unripe fruits in general
Hot water, sugarcane juice, coconut water, milk, coconut milk, mustard oil, sesame oil, coconut oil, buttermilk and yoghurt	Cool drinks

Pitta (Bile)

Favourable	Avoidable
Legumes, brown soya, ragi, wheat, green soya, barley and oats	Millet, rice, corn
Coriander, cumin, turmeric	Dry ginger, mustard, pepper, coriander leaves, fenugreek, saffron, asafoetida, clove, cinnamon and cardamom

Snake gourd, ash gourd, pumpkin, gooseberry, cucumber, cabbage, beans, ladies finger, cauliflower and celery	Brinjal, hot pepper, tomato, egg, fruit, tapioca, spinach, onion, radish, tender mango, garlic, carrot, beetroot and green chilly
Orange, grapes, apple, dates, coconut, pomegranate	Mango, apricot, banana, grapes, berries, pineapple, unripe fruits
Sunflower oil, olive oil, boiled-cold water, sugarcane juice, coconut water, cow's milk, coconut milk, clarified butter and honey	Almond oil, sesame oil, goat's milk, hot water, mustard oil, castor oil, alcohol, buttermilk and yoghurt

Kapha (Mucus)

Favourable	Avoidable
Lentils, green soya, horse gram, rye, rice, barley, wheat, brown gram and corn	Black soya, oats and green peas.
Dry ginger, mustard, coriander leaves, coriander, cumin seed, nutmeg, pepper, asafoetida, fenugreek, clove, saffron, cinnamon	
Snake gourd, asparagus, bitter gourd, drumstick, brussels, sprouts, brinjals, spinach, cabbage, tender mango, gooseberry, carrot, beetroot, green chilly, ash gourd, radish, potato and onion	Cucumber, sweet potato, sweet and juicy vegetables, ladies finger, colocasia, tender jackfruit
Orange, apricot, lemon, berries, pomegranate, apple and pear	Jackfruit, avocado, bananas, grapes, coconut, dates, plums, melon, papaya, sweets, sour and very juicy fruits
Honey, hot water, goat's milk, mustard oil, buttermilk, castor oil, sesame oil, alcohol, sunflower oil	Sugarcane juice, coconut water, milk, coconut milk, clarified butter, yoghurt and coconut oil

About Tastes

Taste	Properties	Action	Disorders by excess use
Sweet	Oily, cold, and heavy	Bulk promoting, vitaliser, tonic, laxative, diuretic, increases mucus and decreases wind and bile	Obesity, anorexia, respiratory disorders, goitre, lymphadenitis, filarial, diabetes, worms etc.
Sour	Oily, hot and heavy	Appetizer, digestive, carminative, useful in anorexia, harmful for semen, increases mucus and bile and reduces wind	Blood disorders, swelling, inflammations, burning sensation, skin diseases, anaemia, hemorrhage, vertigo, defects of vision
Salty	Oily and hot	Heavy, moistening, appetizer, digestive, breaking, expectorant, harmful for semen, increases mucus, bile and reduces wind	Impotency, gray hairs, falling of hairs, hemorrhage, gastritis, erysipelas, skin disorders
Pungent	Rough, dry, hot and light	Mouth cleansing, appetizer, digestive, bulk reducing, anathematic, useful in dyspepsia, increases wind, reduces bile and mucus	Impotency, unconsciousness, vertigo, debility, burning sensation and thirst
Bitter	Rough, dry, cold and light	Appetizer, digestive, anthelmintic, antipyretic, antipoison, increases wind, reduces bile and mucus	Emaciation, debility, vertigo, dryness of mouth, nervous diseases
Astringent	Rough, dry, cold and light	Astringent, absorbent, healing, harmful for semen, increases wind, reduces bile and mucus	Dryness of mouth, cardiac pain, tympanitis, obstruction in channels, impotency, nervous disorders

Prana (elan vital) moves all over the body. Apana helps to eliminate stool, urine etc. In a state of equilibrium Samana maintains drinkables, eatables, smellables, blood, bile, mucus etc. The responsible wind for pulsation, fluttering of eyes, mouth etc. is called Udana. Vyana wind destroys the organs of the body, aggravates the diseases and annihilates the sense of pleasures.

The colour of Prana is molten silver, Apana is red, Samana is reddish, Udana is milky and Vyana is crystal.

Pacaka (Bile) pitta which is located between colon and stomach, helps by its own power in immediate digestion and disintegration of four types of food and drinks. Ranjaka bile located in liver and spleen imparts colour to chyle or plasma. Sadhaka bile located in heart penetrates the mucus lodged in the heart in the form of tames and by doing so it helps in accomplishment of religious virtues, satisfaction of desires, ego etc. Alocaka bile located in the eyes helps in the perception of vision. Bhrajaka bile helps in assimilation of drugs used in the form of massage, sprinkling etc., and helps in manifestation of complexion and aura.

Mucus located in stomach, chest, heart and joints gives sturdiness and compactness to the whole body. Avalambaka mucus located in stomach supports the location of the remaining mucus. Kledaka mucus causes disintegration and paste form of food. Bodhaka mucus located in the tongue helps in the perception of tastes. Tarpaka mucus located in the head causes nourishment of the eyes. Slesaka mucus located in joints helps in cohesiveness of the joints.

Vata (wind) is light, ununctuous, mobile, cooling and gets digested, after it pervades the entire body, non-slimy, rough, subtle, moves fastly, restricts normal movements of stool, urine etc., and it has the power to move speedily.

Its functions are: enthusiasm, respiration, motor activities, maintenance of body tissues, functioning of sense organs.

Bile is subtle, sour, pungent, bitter, hot, associated with unctuousness, acute performance, liquid, ability to spread, yellow, red, sharp. It causes looseness of joints. Functions: digestion, craving for hot things, hunger, thirst, lucidity and clarity of mind, vision, retention of knowledge, courage in making decision and softness of body.

Mucus is sweet, unctuous, soft, cold, stable, smooth, slime, heavy, dense, sluggish, while by nature in the state of proper digestion sweet taste, and improper digestion saline taste. Functions: stability, visidity, healthy reproduction function, strength of joints, forbearance, intelligence, courage, strength, constant nature of mood, healing, storage, roborant and soothing.

Their specific attributes are: wind — roughness, bile—sharpness, mucus—unctuousness.

Ununctuousness etc., associated with heat causes the accumulation of wind which gets aggravated by cold, and alleviated by cold, and alleviated by ununctuousness.

Bile gets accumulated when sharpness etc. are associated with cold; gets aggravated by heat and alleviated by sluggishness etc., associated with cold.

Mucus gets accumulated by unctuousness etc., due to the association of cold; gets aggravated by heat, and alleviated by ununctuousness etc.

By improper food and improper regimens, humours are accumulated. It may happen instantaneously or gradually in appropriate time.

Signs and symptoms of accumulation:

Absence of any peristaltic movement of the intestines

Feeling as if intestines are filled up with something

Reduction in the temperature

Laziness and heaviness in the body

Yellowishness in the body

Finding fault in any good thing without any reason

Channels for spreading humours are periphery, gastro-intestinal tract and vital organs like brain, heart, urinary bladder etc. The skin and tissue elements (hemoglobin fraction of blood) constitute periphery. The diseases are black or white spots on the skin, goitre, pimple, growth in the skin, tumour, anaemia, piles, phantom tumour and oedema.

Gastro-intestinal tract comprises stomach, small intestine, colon and rectum. The diseases are vomiting, diarrhea, bronchitis, asthma, obstinate abdominal diseases, ascites and fever.

Diseases manifested in the 3rd channel (vital organs) are trembling of the body, paralysis, facial paralysis, headache etc.

Wind gets aggravated by fighting with strong person, excessive physical exercise, excessive indulgence in sex, excessive loud speech, fall, running, pressure or injury to the body, fasting, floating, swimming, night awakening, head-load carrying, travelling to distance on elephant, horse, car or cart, intake of food or drinks which are pungent, astringent or bitter in taste, unctuous, light and cold in potency, intake of dried vegetables, dried fish, irregularity in taking food, food before well digestion of the previous meal, suppression of the urge of passing flatus, micturition, defaecation, vomiting, sneezing, eructation and tear and such other factors.

It gets specially aggravated by cold, onset of cloud, wind at the end of summer, in the late night, in the afternoon and after the digestion of food.

Diseases by aggravation of wind: 1. Cracking of nails, 2. Cracking of feet, 3. Pain in foot, 4. Foot drop, 5. Numbness of foot, 6. Club foot, 7. Stiff ankle, 8. Cramps of calf muscle, 9. Sciatica, 10. Jenu Varum, 11. Jenu Valgum, 12. Stiffness and fullness of thigh, 13. Pain and weakness in the thigh, 14. Paraplegia, 15. Prolapse of rectum, 16. Tenesmus (Gudarti), 17. Scrotal pain, 18. Stiffness of penis, 19. Fullness of groin, 20. Pelvic pain, 21. Hard stool, 22. Abdominal distension with constipation, 23. Lameness, kyphosis, 24. Dwarfism, 25. Pain and stiffness in sacroiliac joint, 26. Stiffness of back, 27. Chest pain, 28. Spasmodic abdominal pain, 29. Bradycardia, 30. Tachycardia/palpitation, 31. Rubbing chest pain, 32. Impairment of thoracic movement, 33. Pricking chest pain, 34. Atrophy of arm, 35. Stiffness of neck, 36. Torticollis, 37. Hoarseness of voice, 38. Jaw pain, 39. Lip pain, 40. Eye pain, 41. Toothache, 42. Loose tooth, 43. Dump, 44. Lalling speech, 45. Astringent taste of mouth, 46. Dryness of mouth, 47. Ageusia, 48. Anosmia, 49. Ear- ache, 50. Tinnitus, 51. Hard hearing, 52. Deafness, 53. Ptosis of eyelid, 54. Entropion, 55. Amaurosis, 56. Pain in eyes, 57. Ptosis of eyeballs, 58. Ptosis of eyebrow, 59. Pain in temporal region, 60. Pain in frontal region, 61. Headache, 62. Dandruff, 63. Facial paralysis, 64. Monoplegia, 65. Polyplegia, 66. Hemiplegia, 67. Clonic convulsions, 68. Tonic convulsions, 69. Fainting, 70. Giddiness, 71. Tremor, 72. Yawning, 73. Hiccup, 74. Asthenia, 75. Delirium, excess talk, 76. Dryness, 77. Hardness, 78. Dusky dark appearance, 79. Insomnia, 80. Unstable mind.

Symptoms of aggravation of wind: 1. It gets aggravated at night and is reduced during daytime. There is instantaneous remission of pain. 2. Rigidity and contraction of hands and legs, 3. Spreads acute pain to lumbar region, pelvic region, liver, spleen, back of chest, abdomen, testicle etc. 4. Bad taste in mouth, roughness of the skin and irregularity of power of digestion, emaciation, hyper pigmentation of body, tremor, abnormal pulsation, affinity for hot things, fainting, insomnia, inspired sense, acute pain of bones, depletion of tissue, constipation, flatulence, hyper peristaltic movement, loss of concentration, fear, great and irregular speed.

Treatment for diseases of wind: 1. Fomentation and oleation, 2. Mild elimination, 3. Drugs and diet having sweet, sour and saline taste, 4. Drugs and diet should be hot, 5. Alcohol made of pastries and molasses, 6. Regular intake of medicated enema of unctuous and hot drugs, 7. Leisurely living, 8. Oil, ghee, etc., boiled with drugs that are digestive, stimulant and carminative, 9. Application of hot ointment and hot medicated bath, warm soup and milk.

Bile gets aggravated by anger, grief, fear, exertion, fasting, indigestion leading to acid formation, sexual intercourse, intake of pungent, sour, saline, sharp, hot ingredients that are bad for digestion and acid forming, sesame oil, oil cake, green vegetables, curd, butter, milk, alcoholic preparations, sour fruits etc. It gets specially aggravated by heat, during summer, at the end of rainy season, during midday, and midnight, and at the time of digestion of food.

Symptoms of aggravated bile: Yellow coloration of skin, giddiness, weakness, defective functioning of sense organs, destruction of ojas, desire for cold things, burning sensation, bitter taste in mouth, excessive thirst, fainting, reduced sleep and anger.

Diseases of bile: 1. Burning sensation, 2. Scorching, 3. Burning, 4. Boiling, 5. Fuming, 6. Acid regurgitation, 7. Pyrosis, 8. Internal burning sensation, 9. Burning sensation in shoulder, 10. Excessive temperature, 11. Profuse sweating, 12. Foetid body smell, unpleasant smell, 13. Cracking bodyache, 14. Sloughing of blood, 15. Sloughing of muscles, 16. Burning sensation in the skin, 17. Cracking of the skin, 18. Itching of the skin, 19. Urticaria, 20. Red vesicle formation, 21. Bleeding disorders, 22. Red round patches, 23. Greenish discoloration, 24. Yellowish discoloration, 25. Blue spot, 26. Herpes, 27. Jaundice, 28. Bitter taste of mouth, 29. Metallic odour of mouth, 30. Bad odour of mouth, 31. Excessive thirst, 32. Dissatisfaction, 33. Stomatitis, 34. Pharyngitis, 35. Conjunctivitis, 36. Proctitis, 37. Inflammation of penis, 38. Hemorrhage, 39. Fainting, 40. Greenish or yellowish discoloration of eyes, urine, and stool. Besides these, giddiness, feeling of intoxication, dryness of mouth, delirium, diarrhea, anorexia, fever, desire of cooling things etc.

Treatment for bile diseases: 1. Intake of clarified butter (ghee), 2. Purgation by drugs of sweet and cooling, 3. Drugs and diet having taste of sweet, bitter and pungent, 4. Bath with perfume, 5. External application of camphor and sandal paste, 6. Pearl necklace, 7. Patience, 8. Exposure during early hours of night to moon rays on the roof, 9. Association with friends who are free and informal, 10. Talking to those whose speech is pleasing and sweet, 11. Association with ladies who are informal with camphor perfume and who wear ornaments, 12. Stay in cold house (house below water is good), 13. House (with underground rooms) through which a stream flows, 14. Walk in parks and on the banks of lakes, 15. Sitting on the sand of the lakes having well formed banks and clean water.

Special regimens to alleviate bile: Bank of a lotus pond, a park with sufficient trees, pleasing gestures, milk and clarified butter and purgation.

Mucus gets aggravated by sleep during the daytime, lack of exercise, lazy habits, eating sweets, sour, saline, cold unctuous, heavy, slimy and which obstructs the channels of circulation, food like wheat, sesame, pastry prepared of sesame and its other preparations, curd, milk, alkaline, puddings, sugarcane juice, intake of excess food, eating before previous food is digested and other wrong regimens.

Symptoms of aggravated mucus: Pallor, coldness, flabbiness, obesity, laziness, heaviness, loss of strength of body, obstruction of channels, fainting, excess sleep, drowsiness, dyspnoea, cough, excessive salivation, nausea, loss of digestive power, abnormal function of joints.

It gets specially aggravated by cold, in winter, in spring, in the forenoon, in the evening and soon after eating.

Diseases of mucus: 1. Anorexia, 2. Drowsiness, 3. Excessive sleep, 4. Timidness, 5. Heaviness of the body, 6. Lethargy, 7. Sweet taste in the mouth, 8. Salivation, 9. Mucus expectoration, 10. Excessive excretion of excreta, 11. Weakness, indigestion, 12. Feeling of covering over the heart, 13. Phlegm adhered to throat, 14. Hardening of blood vessels, 15. Goitre, 16. Obesity, 17. Loss of appetite or digestive fire, 18. Urticaria, 19. Pallor, 20. Whiteness of urine, eyes and stool. Besides these, cardiac diseases, itching over the body, excessive horripilation, ineffectiveness of wisdom, vomiting, chronic rhinitis, bronchitis, sensation in lips, throat, tongue, gums, palate, nose, eyes, ears and earlobes.

Treatment for mucus diseases: 1. Administration of emetic and inhalation with sharp drugs, 2. Intake of light and ununctuous food, 3. Exercise, unction, kneading, smoking, medicated gargles, 4. Fat reducing drugs,

5. Fomentation, 6. Intake of old wheat, honey, 7. Old alcoholic drinks and 8. Avoid daytime sleep.

As wind is ununctuous, cold and light, gingili (sesame) oil alleviates wind. Bile is hot, not sweet and sharp; so ghee (clarified butter) alleviates bile. Mucus is unctuous, sweet and sluggish. So honey alleviates it.

AMA AND NIRAMA

Ama: Ama is on the analogy of the production of poison by fermented fluids. If the power usma (factors responsible for digestion and metabolism) is subdued the first dhatu rasa (plasma and chyle) does not get properly digested. Being vitiated, the plasma enters into stomach and small intestine. It is called Ama. In other words Ama is produced as a result of internal action among the exceedingly vitiated humours (one with another).

Symptoms of Nirama Mala: If there is no association of Ama with aggravated wind, there will be no pain during eating, less pain during digestion and more pain after digestion. If there is no association of Ama with vitiated bile, there will be no pain after digestion, less pain during eating, and more pain during digestion. If there is no association of Ama with vitiated mucus, there will be no pain after digestion, less pain during digestion, and more pain soon after eating. If the pain occurs in the reverse order, it must be due to the association of Ama.

If Ama is associated with malas and humours the symptoms are: 1. Obstruction to the channels of circulation, 2. Diminution of strength, 3. Heaviness, anorexia, dumbness, absence of any movement of wind and laziness, 4. Indigestion and spitting of saliva, 5. Obstruction to the passages of stool and urine, 6. Fatigue without effort,

7. Yellow stool, urine, nail, teeth and eyes, 8. Red or black coloration of the above organs, 9. Headache, 10. Drowsiness, 11. Pain in back, bone, lumbar and joints, 12. Oedema in the body, 13. Fever and diarrhea, 14. Tingling sensation, 15. Discoloration, 16. Absence of taste in mouth, and 17. Sneezing.

Symptoms of Sama wind: On the association of wind and Ama, constipation, suppression of the power of digestion, drowsiness, gargling sound in the intestines, pain, oedema, excruciating pain. It moves all over the body and afflicts the entire body. It gets aggravated by administration of ghee, during onset of cloud, at dawn and at night.

Symptoms of Nirama wind: Vitiated wind without Ama is non-slimy and ununctuous. It gives less pain, it gets alleviated by substances having properties opposite to it and by administration of unctuous substances like oil, ghee, muscle fat and bone marrow.

Sama bile: Vitiated bile with ama produces foul smell. It is green or greenish gray. It becomes sour, dense and heavy. It produces acidity and burning sensation in the throat and cardiac region.

Nirama bile: Bile without ama is coppery and yellow. It is excessive hot and pungent and it is unstable. It produces foul smell. It causes relish or appetite, digestion and strength.

Sama mucus: Mucus with ama is turbid, thready and dense. It remains in throat and produces foul smell and suppresses appetite and eructation.

Mucus without ama is foamy, compact, yellowish white, without sticky material and without bad smell.

Treatment of Sama humour: Drugs which are carminative and digestive and simulative, 2. Ununctuous fomentation, 3. Purgative by ununctuous drugs, 4. Vomiting, 5. Inhalation, and 6. Fasting.

Humour of wind is most powerful because, 1. It is all over the body, 2. It maintains its action instantaneously, 3. It acts independently with other humours, 4. It has the power to vitiate remaining humours, 5. It has the ability to penetrate into all parts of the body.

Either one or two or all the three humours get mixed up with the fluid etc., they afflict several organs. For wind's migration to the location of bile, the treatment prescribed for bile should be adopted for the wind. For bile's migration to the place of mucus, the patient should be treated on the line of treatment for aggravated mucus. For mucus's migration to the place of wind the line of treatment of wind should be adopted.

Due to the affliction of wind to the heart the patient is given ununctuous drugs for vomiting. But if wind migrates to stomach (location of mucus) ordinary vomiting is enough.

Time of vitiation of blood is determined on the basis of aggravation of humours by which it is afflicted.

Different pains caused by aggravation of wind: 1. Needle pierced pain, 2. Skin excised pain, 3. Pain as if organ is beaten with a stick, 4. Pain as if organ is cut by a weapon or by incision, 5. Pain by extension of a contracted organ, 6. Pain by churning of the inside of an ulcer, 7. Pain as if something is thrown out, 8. Pain by application of paste, 9. Pain by complete burning of the organ, 10. Breaking pain, 11. Pain by striking a stone, 12. Pain by incision through nail, 13. Pain by pulling out something from the body, 14. Pain with shivering, 15. Colic pain pierced by sharp pointed weapon, 16. Pain of dislocation, 17. Pain as if surface of the ulcer is breaking at different places, 18. Pain caused by arrest of movement, 19. Pain as if something is fitted up by force, 20. Numbness, 21. Pain by folding an organ from several places, 22. Pain when a part of the organ is pierced by sharp rounded weapon, 23. Appearance of different types of pain without any perceptible cause, 24. Frequent appearance of pain.

Pain of vitiated wind: 1. Burning sensation in a part of organ, 2. Pain as if something is sucked, 3. Burning all over the body, 4. Pain as hot smoke coming out of the body, 5. Pain as if entire body is covered with hot charcoal and cooked, 6. Increase in temperature, 7. Pain as alkali spread over an ulcer.

Pain by vitiation of mucus: 1. Itching, 2. Heaviness, 3. Feeling as if something is applied externally, 4. Loss of pain, 5. Rigidity, 6. Cold in touch.

MALAS (EXCRETA)

Faeces causes a sense of compactness of the body. It is an excellent agent for the sustenance of strength and factors responsible for digestion and metabolism. Urine fills up the bladder. Sweat gives stickiness to the body. Menstrual blood promotes excellence of the organs of the woman's body and it is responsible for conception.

Signs of diminution of humours: 1. Excessive administration of elimination therapies, 2. Suppression of manifested urges, 3. Improper exercise, 4. Excessive walking, 5. Mental worries.

Diminution of wind: 1. Absence of excitement, 2. Loss of speech, 3. Unconsciousness, 4. Absence of sensation, 5. Irregular movement of the limbs.

Diminution of bile: 1. Loss of temperature, 2. Absence of digestive power and metabolism, and 3. Loss of lustre.

Diminution of mucus: 1. Burning sensation inside the body, 2. Ununctuousness, 3. Feeling of emptiness in colon and stomach including small intestine, 4. Looseness of joints.

Diminution of Rasa: 1. Pain in the cardiac region, 2. Dryness of throat, 3. Feeling of emptiness, and 4. Excessive thirst.

Diminution of hemoglobin fraction of the blood: 1. Roughness of skin, 2. Looseness of veins.

Diminution of muscle tissue: 1. Dryness, 2. Emaciation, 3. Roughness, 4. Pain and looseness in thigh, hip joints, axilla, buttocks, hips, genital organ, and 5. Mandibular eminence in the face.

Diminution of fat: 1. Enlargement of spleen, 2. Emptiness of joints, 3. Roughness, 4. Desire of taking fatty things (meat etc.).

Diminution of bone tissue: 1. Pain in bones, 2. Cracking of nails and teeth.

Diminution of bone marrow: 1. Diminution of quantity of semen, 2. Breaking pain in phalanges, 3. Feeling of emptiness in the bones, 4. Pain in bones.

Diminution of semen: 1. Pain in genital organ, 2. Pain in the testicles, 3. Inability in the performance of sexual act, 4. Ejaculation of semen after a long time, 5. Ejaculate small quantity of semen, 6. More blood with semen during ejaculation.

Diminution of faeces: 1. Pain in cardiac region and sides of the chest, 2. Ejaculation of flatus with sound, 3. Upward movement of the wind from the lower abdomen.

Diminution of urine: 1. Pain in the urinary bladder, 2. Elimination of less quantity of urine.

Diminution of sweat: 1. Numbness in hair follicles, 2. Roughness of skin, 3. Unctuous ointment applied gets dried up immediately, 4. Absence of sweating, 5. Roughness in touch.

Diminution of menstrual blood: 1. Pain in female genital, 2. Absence of any bleeding during menstruation, 3. Less amount of bleeding during menstruation.

Diminution of breast milk: 1. Looseness of breast, 2. Absence of lactation, 3. Loss of lactation.

LINE OF TREATMENT FOR DIMINUTION

Diminished humours, dhatus, excreta and strength can be re-equipped by taking such diet and drinks which increase the quantity of these elements. Desired diet and drink helps in overcoming the diminution of respective elements.

Light food with astringent, pungent and bitter tastes is suggested for patient suffering from diminution of wind.

Different pastries with sesame, sour buttermilk and yoghurt can be given to the patients for diminution of bile.

To cure the diminution of mucus, meat of buffalo, pig and goat, jaggery, heavy food, more milk and yoghurt.

Sugarcane, clarified butter, meat soup, honey, jaggery, water, blood and gruel are given for the patient of diminution of rasa.

Grapes, pomegranate with fat and salt are suggested for diminution of blood.

To cure semen diminution, give eggs of peacock, cock, swan, duck and other birds of marshy land and aquatic.

Curd (yoghurt) and different kinds of vegetables can be given to improve faeces diminution.

Thin gruel, sugarcane juice, milk with jaggery are good to cure urine diminution.

Diminution of sudation can be treated by massage, alcoholic drink, sleep, stay in a room free from wind and covering the body with thick warm sheets.

To cure diminution of menstruation give pungent food, sour and saline taste, sour drinks, food that can cause burning sensation and salty fruits and vegetables and post-prandial drinks.

There are three kinds of therapies: Spiritual therapy, reasoning therapy (physical and chemical property) and psychic therapy.

Spiritual therapy: Spiritual energy massage, incantation, chanting of mantras, wearing of talisman and gems, auspicious recitation, offerings, gifts, oblations, observance of spiritual rules, chanting of auspicious hymns, pilgrimage, fasting, atonement and paying obeisance to gods.

Reasoning therapy: Proper ingredients in diet and medicine, considering the taste etc. are the therapy based on reasoning (physical and chemical property).

The **psychic therapy** consists in withdrawal of mind from harmful objects and practice of intellectual performance, patience and spiritual knowledge and spiritual energy massage.

Other classifications are: 1. Internal cleansing, 2. External cleansing, and 3. Surgical therapy. While entering into the body the drugs and diet which cleanse either by elimination or by nourishment is called internal cleansing.

Incision, excision, blood letting by leeches etc. constitute surgical therapy.

LAND

There are two types of land to be considered in Ayurveda. 1. The land where the patient lives, 2. Physique (body) of the individual.

The patients live in three types of land. 1. Marshy land, 2. Forest, and 3. Land in general having mixed character.

Marshy land: It is full of rivers, lakes, mountains, lotus, lilies, having several kinds of birds, pigs, buffaloes, big trees, full of flowers and many vegetation and fruits. It has rice fields.

The inhabitants of this land suffer from diseases of wind and mucus, less power of digestion, short span of life and less strength. They are fatty, bulky with mobile breasts and belly. So for their happiness their diet and drinks should be that which do not obstruct the channels of circulation, unctuous, sour, light and which stimulate the power of digestion.

Forest: Cloudless sky, sand and irregular land surrounded with trees. There are deer, donkey, ass, cattle etc. and also wild animals. Water will be less but healthy.

People are less fat, sturdy and hardworking. They have beautiful and compact body and less desires, long span of life. They suffer from diseases of wind. Their diet and drinks should be nourishing, heavy, unctuous and liquid.

Land of general nature: There will be equal quantity of rain, cold, heat and wind. The humours are in equilibrium. So it is healthy to live.

One who resorts to diet, sleep and other activities that are conducive to the characteristic features of land does not get afflicted by its evil effects.

Land suitable for collection of herbs:

Land having stones, soil, stable and bluish black or black in colour, having thick trees and vegetation is earthy element land.

Windy element land is unctuous, with uneven colour and thin trees with less of sap.

Fiery element land has different colour, light, sandy less trees with yellow colour.

The land of ether element is soft, even, free from clouds, water with imperceptible taste, surrounded by emaciated trees with bluish-black colour and big mountains.

Root, leaf, bark, latex, flower and fruit should be collected in the beginning of rainy season, autumn, winter, spring and summer respectively. Collect the cooling medicines in winter and hot medicines in summer. Cooling medicines collected in winter are impregnated with cooling effect of the earth and so are extremely sweet, unctuous and cooling in nature.

Collect the pungent drugs from earth dominated and water dominated land.

Collect the emetic drugs from wind and fire dominated land.

Humours alleviating drugs should be collected from ether dominated land.

DIFFERENT NATURE OF CONSTITUTION (PRAKRITI)

Humours constituting nature of constitution are: 1. Semen including sperm and ovum, 2. Food of the pregnant, 3. Regimens during pregnancy, 4. Condition prevailing inside the uterus and 5. Seasonal effect. Nature is caused by humours inherent in sperm and ovum immediately before the conception. Nature caused by wind, bile and mucus are inferior, mediocre and superior respectively. Prakriti caused by humours of equilibrium is the best among all. Prakriti caused by two, e.g., wind-bile, bile-mucus, mucus-wind are disposable ones. Prakriti which are manifested at the time of conception are incapable of afflicting the individual.

Windy constitution (Vata Prakriti): 1. Body is rough to touch and thin, 2. Black complexion, 3. Poor voice, 4. Short stature and less voice, 5. Quick in attempt and quick in giving it up, 6. Likes delicious food, 7. Talkative, 8. Wakes for a long time, 9. Inability to walk along, 10. Poor disposition, 11. Long nails, 12. Dreams of moving in the sky, 13. Cracks in the skin, sole and palm and 14. Fickleness of mind.

Bile constitution (Pitta Prakriti): 1. Body hot, white, tender and loose, 2. Excess of thirst and hunger, 3. Reddish, soft and thin hair, 4. Power of digestion and metabolism is sharp, 5. Early wrinkles and graying hair, 6. Foul smell from axilla, 7. Coppery colour of eyes, 8. Unctuous and plump body, 9. Likes different types of work and food, 10. Less small hair on the body, 11. Likes flattering, 12. Likes bitter taste and 13. More sweating.

Mucus constitution (Kapha Prakriti): 1. Unctuous and plump body, 2. Good complexion and sense organs, 3. Strong body, 4. Good patience, 5. Slow walk, 6. Less of foul smell, presence of good smell in the body, 7. Good memory, 8. Less talkative, 9. Less diseases in summer and hot countries.

Constitution of humour equilibrium (Sama Prakriti): 1. Mixed coloration of the body, 2. Compact limbs, 3. Small hairs of the body, deep rooted without crack, 4. Loves ladies, 5. Can carry heavy weight and 6. Endowed with luxurious life.

Sixteen types of prakriti: 7 satwik, 6 rajasik and 3 tamasik.

Process of life: 1. Tenderness of age, 2. Growth, 3. Aura, 4. Intellect, 5. Skin, 6. Characteristic features, 7. Semen, 8. Forceful attempt, 9. Wisdom, 10. Functions of the motor organs.

Table of characteristics of individuals

Satwik

1.	Sharing the traits of Brahma	1. Purity and love for truth, 2. Sincerity in effort, 3. Pray to God and preceptor, 4. Respect guests, 5. Endeavour to acquire knowledge.
2.	Sharing traits of Mahendra	1. Great fame and courage, 2. Obedience, 3. Constant devotion to scriptural study, 4. Proper maintenance of servants.
3.	Sharing traits of Varuna	1. Like cold things, 2. Tolerance, 3. Coppery colour, 4. Greenish colour of hair, 5. Pleasing talks.
4.	Sharing traits of Kubera	1. Work as moderator, 2. Tolerability, 3. Acquiring of wealth, 4. Great power to deliver goods.
5.	Sharing traits of Gandharva	1. Like scents and garlands, 2. Desire for dance and music, 3. Like to move about.
6.	Sharing traits of Yama	1. Observance of propriety of action, 2. Initiation of strong action, 3. Fearlessness, 4. Memory and parity, 5. Freedom from attachment, illusion, fear and envy.
7.	Sharing traits of Rishi	1. Devotion to penance and sacred rituals, 2. Celibacy, oblation to fire and study, 3. Marital and spiritual knowledge.

Rajasik

1.	Sharing traits of Asura	1. Endowed with wealth, 2. Terrifying, brave, cruel and envious, 3. Like enjoyments only, 4. Like to satisfy belly.
2.	Sharing traits of Bird	1. Excessive indulgence in sex, 2. Frequent eating, 3. Anger and instability.
3.	Sharing traits of Snake	1. Sharpness, deceptiveness, cowardice, cruelty and intelligence, 2. Fickleness in movement and eating.

4.	Sharing traits of Rakshasa	1. One sided thinking, 2. Anger and envy, 3. Absence of religious mind, 4. Like self-praise.
5.	Sharing traits of Pisaca	1. Left out food eating, 2. Sharpness, 3. Like bravery, 4. Like women, 5. Shamelessness.
6.	Sharing traits of Pretas	1. Do not like to share enjoyment, 2. Laziness, 3. Miserable disposition, 4. Jealousy, 5. Greediness, 6. Do not like to give charity.

Tamasik

1.	Sharing traits of animal	1. Lack of intelligence, 2. Sluggishness, 3. Indulgence in sex during dreams, 4. Disobedience.
2.	Sharing traits of fish	1. Instability, 2. Lack of wisdom, 3. Cowardice, 4. Like water, 5. Mutual distribution of each other.
3.	Sharing traits of vegetation	1. Like to stay only at one place, 2. Like only eating, 3. Absence of mental faculty, religion, 4. Desire and wealth.

Chapter 3

IMPORTANCE OF MATTERS (DRAVYAS)

Matters (Dravyas) are two—manifested and unmanifested. After the process of combination of five subtle tanmatras (primary elements), the matter becomes manifested. In the absence of combination of five subtle tanmatras the matter remains unmanifested. As the treatment is initiated on the basis of manifested matter, only the manifested matter will be described here.

Drugs play the role of sweet music and they are differently classified. 1. As creeper and tree, 2. Immovable as metals, minerals and vegetable kingdom, 3. Movables as animals, birds, etc., 4. Kanda (rhizome) root, fruits and flowers, 5. Sterile and fertile, and 6. Domesticated and wild.

The living creatures have four sources of origin. 1. In the mother's womb covered by amniotic membrane, 2. From egg, 3. Out of sweat or moist heat, and 4. By perforating the earth (including vegetables).

Drugs are called earthy, watery, fiery, windy and ethery. But they are classified as having heating effect and cooling effect.

According to therapeutic effect drugs are classified: 1. Care by eliminating the humours, 2. Care by alleviating the humours. Stable drugs are available on or inside the earth. They come out by penetrating the earth.

Drugs on or inside the earth are: mud, lime, sand, stone, salt, alkaline collected from caves, collyrium, red ochre, metals, pyrite, gold, mercury, gems and jewels, broken pieces of earthen pots.

Drugs that come out by penetrating the earth are: trees having fruits without flowers, plants die when fruits are mature, creepers and trees with flowers and fruits, roots, leaves, fruits, flowers, barks, aqueous extract or heartwood, juice, latex, milk of plants, oil, gum, stalk and rhizomes.

Movable Dhatus (matters) are: 1. Skin, blood, meat, fat, bone, bone marrow and semen, 2. Milk, bile, 3. Honey, beeswax, stools and urine, 4. Gorocana solidified ox-bile (viscera), 5. Hair, small hair, ligament, horn, tooth and hoof, 6. Kostha abdominal and thoracic viscera, 7. Testicles and feather.

Earthy drugs are heavy, gross, stable, with more smell. Such drugs cause heaviness, stability, compactness and plumpness.

Watery drugs are liquid, cold, heavy, unctuous, sluggish and dense. Having more taste they cause unctuousness, obstruction to channels of circulation, stickiness, happiness and cohesiveness.

Fiery drugs are unctuous, sharp, hot, non-slimy and subtle. Having more colour they cause burning sensation, aura and complexion of the body.

Windy drugs are ununctuous, non-slimy and light. Having tactual attributes they cause roughness, subtlety, movement and feeling of exhaustion without effort.

Sky drugs are subtle, non-slimy and light. Having more sound they cause porosity and lightness. They have unmanifested taste.

Emetic drugs are dominated by wind and fire and by nature they have the tendency to move upwards.

Purgative drugs are dominated by earth and water, and by nature, they have the tendency to move downwards.

Astringent (bowel binding) drugs are dominated by wind.

Nourishing drugs are of water. The drugs that alleviate humours are of ether. Drugs dominated by earth are promoters of strength. Digestive drugs stimulate digestion of undigested food or metabolic byproduct (deepana).

Drugs help in maturing digestion (Pacana) of undigested food materials or metabolic byproduct.

Helping digestive fire drugs are dominated by fire, and they cause digestion and metabolic transformation of Ama (toxin). These drugs being dominated by wind and fire possess hot property and therefore become pungent in taste after digestion.

Promoting digestive (deepana) drugs have sweet taste and cooling property. Drugs that stimulate digestive fire but do not help in digestion of ama (undigested food material or metabolic byproduct).

Fasting is Pacana (maturing digestive fire) not deepana (stimulating digestion). By elimination therapies, bloodletting, oleation and fasting, the digestive fire gets diminished.

Drugs helpful in digestion cleanse the channels of circulation vitiated by mucus. These drugs help in metabolic transformation of tissue elements (Dhatu).

Deepana drugs stimulate the digestive fire, but do not help in digestion of ama (toxin), e.g., clarified butter.

Drugs that do not stimulate digestive fire, but cause metabolic transformation or immature digestive and metabolic products are called Pacana.

Drug that causes downward movement of wind is called anuloma drug. Drug that alleviates the vitiated humour but does not eliminate or vitiate the normal humours is called Samana drug.

Drugs which eliminate the excreta and are digested after disintegrating the solid state are called Sramsana.

Drugs that eliminate both solid and disintegrated excreta through downward tract are called Bhedana.

Drugs that eliminate both digested and indigested excreta by dissolving through downward tract are called Virecana (Purging).

Drug that eliminates the indigested mucus and bile through upward tract is called Vamana (Vomiting).

Drug that by force uproots the adhered humours is called Chedana.

Drug, which, because of its heating nature, works as digestive stimulant and carminative, causes constipation is called Grahi.

Drug that is light for digestion, because of its astringent taste causes constipation is called Stambhana.

Drug which destroys the process of aging and diseases is called Rasayana.

Drug that causes excitement and passionate desire for woman is called Vajikara.

Drug that increases the quantity of semen is called Sukrala, e.g., aswagandha, musali, sarkara, and satavari.

A beautiful woman induces the ejaculation of semen. Kshudra (a kind of fruit) causes actual ejaculation, Jatiphala (nutmeg) increases the power of retention of semen, Kaliga seed (seed of a plant) the quantity of semen.

Drug that enters through thin and subtle channels is called Sukshma.

Drug that pervades the whole body before being digested is called Vyavayi. Vikasi drugs loosen the ligaments of joints, cause slackness of hands and legs and separate them.

Madakari drugs are effective in destroying wisdom. Pramathi drugs by their own potency eliminate the humours in the body.

The examples of different categories mentioned above are given below:

Deepana – Chitraka

Pacana – Nagakesara

Samana – Guduci

Anuloma – Haritaki (Anuloma drug causes downward movement of wind)

Sramsana – Krtamala

Bhedana – Katurohini

Recana – Trivrta

Vamana – Madonaphala

Chedana – water & honey

Grahi – cumin

Stambhana – Vatsaka

Rasayana – Guggulu

Vajikara – milk, mosa, talamuli, satavari

Sukshma – Saindhava and honey

Vyavayi – Ahiphena

Vikasi – Kramuka

Madakari – Sura

Yogavahi – Visa

Pramathi – Marica

Abhisyandi – yoghurt (Abhiṣyandi drug obstructs the channels of circulation carrying rasa (plasma) and produces heaviness in the body)

Rasa (taste): The sources of taste, guna (attribute) and karma (action) are innumerable. Mainly there are six tastes: sweet, sour, saline, bitter, pungent and astringent. They are located in six categories of matter (elements) and in the reverse order they are more powerful in nature:

earth and water – sweet; earth and fire – sour;
water and fire – saline; wind and fire – pungent;
wind and ether – bitter; earth and wind – astringent.

Sweet is ascertained by unctuousness, deliciousness, sense of satisfaction, delightfulness, softness and stickiness in the tongue, mouth, palate, throat while the substance is in the mouth.

Sour is ascertained by relish, salivation, setting of teeth on edge and clarity of mouth.

Saline is ascertained by purgation, stickiness, burning sensation, moistness and lightness.

Pungent is ascertained by pinching pain, burning sensation, cutting pain, exudation of watery fluid of mouth, nose and eyes.

Bitter weakens the preparation and causes non-sliminess, delightfulness and dryness.

Astringent causes looseness of joints and produces cooling, rigidity and softness.

Sweet, sour and saline are cooling as they produce unctuousness and stickiness.

Astringent, bitter and pungent are heating.

When wind is aggravated, pungent, bitter and astringent are contraindicated. In bile, pungent, sour and saline are contraindicated. In aggravated mucus, sweet, sour and saline are contraindicated.

Generally sweet aggravates mucus; but old rice, old barley, old wheat, honey and sugar are exceptions.

Sour aggravates bile. But pomegranates, Amalaka are exceptions. Salt generally is unwholesome for eyesight. But rock salt is an exception. Bitter and pungent are exceedingly non-aphrodisiac and aggravate wind. But amrita, patola, ginger etc. are exceptions. Astringent is cooling; but abhaya is an exception.

Pungent, sour and saline are hotter in potency. Bitter, astringent and sweet are cold in potency. Astringent is heavier than saline. Sweet is heavier than astringent, sour is light for digestion and pungent is lighter than sour. Bitter is the lightest.

If all tastes are taken in equal quantity, then the final product becomes sour. If sour is excluded, then the final is pungent. If pungent is also excluded the taste is saline. When pungent, sour and saline are excluded the taste becomes sweet. If bitter and astringent are equal, it will be bitter.

There are twenty attributes: cold, ununctuous, sluggish, light, hot, unctuous, sharp, heavy, slime, non-slime, smooth, rough, hard, soft, liquid, dense, stable, mobile, gross and subtle.

Tastes and humours

Tastes that alleviate wind do not alleviate if there is predominance of attributes of ununctuousness, lightness and coldness in drugs. Tastes that alleviate bile do not do so if there is predominance of sharpness, heat and lightness in the drugs. Tastes that alleviate mucus do not do so if there is predominance of ununctuousness, heaviness, and coldness in the drugs.

Vipaka (taste that emerges after digestion) is of three types — sweet, sour and pungent. Taste that emerges after digestion of sweet and saline tastes is sweet. Vipaka of sour taste is sour. Vipaka of pungent, bitter and astringent is generally pungent.

During the process of digestion of a substance if the attributes of water and earth are excessively manifested the vipaka becomes sweet. During the process of digestion of a substance if fire, wind and ether are manifested in excess the vipaka becomes pungent.

Definition of Vipaka: The taste that emerges in the drug or articles of food by their interaction with digestive enzymes at the end of the process of digestion is called Vipaka.

The factor that is responsible for the manifestation of useful or harmful effects of a drug which is exceedingly useful or harmful is called Prabhava or specific action. The specific action which is manifested in a drug in spite of its similarity with others in taste is called Prabhava.

Cure of poisoning by administration of poison, cure of poisoning and alleviation of all three humours by kasa marda and cure of the serious type of scorpion poisoning by blowing of air impregnated with a mantra into the ear of the patient are the examples of Prabhava (specific action). The magnificent effect of jewels, talisman, mantras and religious rituals is manifested because of their prabhava.

Examination of time/day and night, fortnight, season etc.

Time regulates the phenomena in the world, regulates the phenomena in the morning and evening of the universe and regulates all types of phenomena. Time has its body or unit quantity in the form of year. Its limbs are various seasons. Depending upon the movement of the sun year is divided and subdivided into day, night (second, minute, hour), unit of 15 days depending upon the appearance and disappearance of the moon, month, season, solstice, year and unit of 12 years.

Due to the disturbance in the atmosphere by its rays sun produces cold, heat and rain and it causes seasonal vibrations: late winter, spring, summer, rainy, autumn and early winter are the six seasons. The year is divided into 2, 3, 6 and 12. According to solstice 2, according to rain, cold and heat 3, according to season 6, according to months 12.

To facilitate the comprehension of accumulation of humours and administration of elimination therapies, six divisions of the year (season) are the best.

Late winter, spring and summer constitute northern solstice. During this period, the strength of human being is taken away as the sun and the wind become exceedingly sharp, hot and ununctuous. They take away the cooling attributes from the earth. Bitter, astringent and pungent become more prominent gradually. So northern solstice is heating, period of absorption by nature.

Rainy season, autumn and early winter constitute southern solstice which is elimination period and impregnates the human being with strength. Due to cooling nature moon is powerful, and the power of sun is less. The cloud, rain and wind have cooling effects. The food and drugs are more ununctuous. Sour, saline and sweet are powerful during this period. The living beings acquire considerable energy and cows etc. produce more milk. On the basis of cooling and moistness the wind regulates the activities of the living beings.

The strength in whole winter is superior and in summer and rainy it is inferior. During spring and autumn the strength is mediocre.

Humour of wind gets accumulated in summer, aggravated in rainy and alleviated in autumn. Bile accumulates in rainy, aggravates in autumn, and alleviates in early winter. Mucus accumulates in late winter, aggravates in spring and alleviates in summer.

Regimens of seasons

Early winter: The sky becomes smoky, less dust in the foggy atmosphere. Due to cold wind the sun is less hot, tingling sensation in teeth and horripilation. The earth bears beautiful flowers, more energy among elephants, goats, buffaloes, horses, cows and pigs. Fields look beautiful with blue grains and paddy. All rasas become sweet in Vipaka. Wind and mucus get accumulated. Mucus does not get aggravated in late winter, but gets further accumulated by heavy and unctuous food. It gets soon aggravated only in spring as it gets liquefied due to the hot sun. Due to summer it immediately gets alleviated. In strong men digestive enzymes become powerful as from outside cold covers it. By insufficient food, digestive enzymes being stimulated by wind consume tissue element (Dhatu). Hence men consume more sweet, sour and saline food.

As nights are longer one feels more hunger in the morning. So breakfast should be a little early. As massage alleviates wind, one should have oil massage including the head.

Practise daily yoga and exercises with experts. Knead the body with feet appropriately. Apply oil on head after massage of the body with separate oil as head is superior. If the same oil after body massage is used for head, one loses the virtues and gets inauspiciousness. Kneading with legs after smearing oil is stimulant of digestion and metabolism, and promotes semen, aura and energy and cleanses the ears.

Unction of the body by nourishing drugs promotes complexion and cures itching, obstinate skin diseases and removes excreta. So in the beginning and at the end of exercises apply paste for this purpose. Baking of back in the sun rays is better. Enjoy the heat of the fire from the front. Enjoy heavy and hot food and get fumigated. Women having bulky thighs, breasts and buttocks, strong sexual passion, pleasing, youthful, fumigated with incense and saffron and having warm physique take away the cold. One who dwells in a charcoal-heated house, or underground room or house constructed of earth does not get afflicted with illness caused by the roughness of the cold. In winter, one can take aphrodisiac drugs and indulge in sex as much as he/she likes.

Late winter (Sisara): One should adopt more particularly the regimens of early winter. In winter diseases of wind and mucus afflict human beings for which oil, garlic and linnets are useful. Enjoying with pleasing women is also good.

Spring (Vasant): Spring brings blue leaves and the sound of cuckoo. The god of sex has overwhelming effect during this season. The atmosphere is full of fragrance of flowers. The intoxicated bees roam around the flowers for honey. The earth appears as if in a jubilant mood. It is doubled by the effect of the wind from hills. Mucus is aggravated. Forests are also very beautiful. Due to mucus nausea and suppression of digestion are the main diseases. Mucus gets alleviated after onset of summer. During spring heavy and cold things, sleeping during daytime, unctuous, sour, and sweet food should be avoided. To overcome the aggravated mucus: 1. Emesis with drugs that are sharp in quality, 2. Strong inhalation therapy, 3. Light and ununctuous food, 4. Exercises, unction and kneading, diet, old barley, old wheat, honey etc.

After bath smear the body with paste of camphor, sandal paste, kumkum; drink mango juice served by passionately attached women. This drink is like cardiac tonic. Drakshasav, Abhayarishata etc. can be taken. Water boiled with ginger and with honey is very good. In spring rainwater is also good. Stay in the midday in gardens and parks with flowers of fragrance listening interesting stories and music.

Summer: In summer, pungent is more manifested. Water undergoes Katupaka due to ununctuousness and sharpness of sun rays. So mucus gets alleviated and wind gets accumulated. This wind gets aggravated during rainy season by the impact of clouds and the wind and gets alleviated in autumn due to hot rays of sun.

In summer the sun is sharp and wind blowing from southwest is pleasing. In summer avoid saline, pungent and sour, exercise and exposure to sun. Eat excessive sweet, light, unctuous, cold and liquid, diluted corn flour, ghee, rice, milk, and pastries of wheat with Saindhava.

Water soaking fragrant flowers, making cold, adding camphor. Drink buffalo milk adding sugar and making cold by exposure to moon and stars. Walk in forest where there are trees, creepers and bunches of grapes.

In houses put curtains sprinkling fragrant cold water and hang bundles of mangoes etc. On the bed also soft leaves of lotus, banana, utpala and also with beautiful flowers.

During midday relax in the house having fountains or streams of water inside it. At night sleep on the roof exposed to the moon rays.

Eat mangoes; avoid dry vegetables and leafy vegetables. Diet should be wheat, rice, sugar, buttermilk, milk-water with sugar. Coconut water is very good. Wear white dress.

Rainy: Sky with clouds and rain; water around the earth. Intoxicating wind in all directions; earth filled with warm insects and green-blue tender plants, flooded with water, full of germinated plants, music of the birds; dear and peacocks are happy with sound of the clouds, lotus gets withered, resonance from the caves and services of mountains with full of greenish blue vegetation make the nature more beautiful. Wind gets aggravated as the earth becomes moist, the moisture inside the body also increases. The herbs become reduced in potency. Because of the heat of the earth and because of sour Vipaka of water the power of digestion is suppressed. So fomentation, massage, sleep in free from wind, sex with pleasing and white coloured lady are good. Gradually reduce exercise. Use pungent, sour and alkaline for alleviation of wind and mucus. Diet should be old barley, old wheat, old rice, curd etc. in sufficient quantity. Yoghurt and buttermilk with rock salt is good in correcting the defects in digestive power. Thin buttermilk mixed with powder of some herbs (ginger, rock salt) should be used. Cold water after boiling should be used for drinking. But when there is no rain unboiled water is also good. Don't sleep during daytime. Avoid heavy food, water from river, sexual intercourse, roasted corn flour and exposure to sun.

Autumn: Clouds are beautiful like sunstone. Moon rays are strong, unctuous, clean and more pleasing. Water in the rivers slowly reduces as if a bashful girl of fifteen reluctantly exposes her thighs during her first sexual intercourse. The body adapted to rains and cold is exposed to the hot sun in autumn. So bile accumulated during rains gets vitiated in autumn.

For alleviation of aggravated bile use ghee and eatables of bitter, sweet and astringent taste. Sour predominates in autumn. Purgation, bloodletting are good. Eat light food with honey. Boiled milk with sugar is good. At night expose to moon rays. Sexual intercourse with blackish lady. Use haritaki with honey regularly. For bath, drink and washing use water exposed to the sun in daytime and to the moon at night, which is detoxicated by the effect of star canopus (Agastya). It is cooling, clean and free from all defects.

Don't expose to dew and to the sun. Avoid curd (yoghurt), oil, sleeping during the daytime and also wind from the east. The well-being of life is determined by the amount of sleep during Jyestha and Asadha, quantity of food during Pausha and Magha, and quantity of water during autumn.

Consume all tastes habitually daily. But according to the season certain tastes should be taken in excess.

Transitional phase of season: During transitional period, gradually give up prescriptions of the previous season and resort to the measures prescribed for the consecutive season. If the regimens of the ending season are abruptly given up or if the regimens of the consecutive season are suddenly resorted to, they may give rise to diseases because of unwholesomeness.

One who has nourished tissue elements and equilibrium of digestion and metabolism, who is free from worry and diseases, who is happy, should have desire to enjoy in the appropriate time with young lady and should have intercourse with her according to the prescriptions in the scriptures. During spring and autumn sexual intercourse is permitted on third days. In rainy and summer once in a fortnight (about 9 days total) and with onset of winter sexual intercourse is permitted as much as one desires (may be all 120 days).

Do intercourse at night during winter; in summer in the daytime, in rainy during thunders, in spring both in day and night and during autumn when one is excited.

The invariable desires are: 1. Food, 2. Drinking, 3. Sleep and 4. Sex. Without food the tissue elements burn. Without water blood is reduced. Sleeplessness causes many diseases, and without sex eyesight is afflicted. So these desires should be satisfied appropriately.

Humours accumulated in winter should be eliminated in spring; that accumulated in summer be eliminated in rainy; that accumulated in rainy be eliminated as soon as rains are over. By doing so one can overcome diseases and pain.

Management of epidemics (contagious)

1. Avoid use of such drugs as are devoid of taste and potency. 2. Use only such drugs and water as are grown and collected in appropriate seasons. 3. Perform religious rites and offer prayer to the gods, cows and preceptor etc. 4. Perform penance, sacrifice, rituals for peace, oblation to fire, auspicious invocation, fasting, study of religious scriptures, observance of spiritual rules, meditation and purification, and 5. Abstinence of sense organs from their objects.

One who inhabits in such places — having lot of water, crocodile and fish, where water is alkaline, or sweet, having many rivers or streams flowing through poisonous trees or less quantity of water just descending from mountain — suffers from many diseases and the span of life is short. Headache, bronchitis, asthma, emesis and fever including serious epidemic diseases occur even in unpolluted land, if the air which flows over it has come after passing through a place having poisonous trees, flowers etc. Avoid such places.

Regimen of the day

Get up early morning. After ablution dress the hair, brush teeth with stick of 6" (15 cm) having thickness of little finger. Collect the stick from trees having latex and bitter and astringent taste. Before cutting the tooth stick offer prayer, "Oh tree! Give me life and fame, power of speech, offspring, cattle, wealth, spiritual power, wisdom and intellect." Chew the tip of the tooth stick to brush the teeth and scrap the tongue to remove the bad taste and accumulation of excreta. Mouth becomes non-slimy and light. By gargling mucus gets eliminated and it helps to eliminate excreta. Wash the face with cold water by which bleeding from different parts of the body (Rakta pitta), dryness of mouth, blue mole and appearance of white spots on the face can be cured. Wash mouth with warm pungent water. It eliminates mucus and wind, and cures unctuousness in the face and diseases of mouth.

After food chew betel leaf which is sharp and hot, which alleviates mucus and wind and which cures mouth diseases. Do unction (ubtan) massage. It alleviates mucus and promotes fat, semen etc., increases blood, promotes strength and complexion and alleviates humours. To overcome aging and exertion of body habitual massage is very useful. Massage promotes eyesight, happiness, nourishment, longevity and health. It cures skin diseases and produces sturdiness of the legs. The tissue elements increase in quantity by oil massage.

Bath

For bath use lukewarm water to increase strength. Using hot water for head is not good as it takes away the strength and is harmful for hair and eyesight. Rub the body and head with towel.

In winter wear silk dresses. In summer wear cloth impregnated with juice of astringent trees. In rainy season use white cloth by which the complexion of the body increases. It alleviates itches and skin diseases. In winter using colour silk (red or other) alleviates wind and mucus. Cloth impregnated with decoction of astringent trees promotes intellect; and by its cooling effect it alleviates bile. So use such clothes in summer. White gives pleasure and prevents heat and cold. So use it in rainy season.

Unction over the body with fragrant paste and then ointments of saffron, sandal etc. should be smeared over the body. These ointments have heating property. So use them in winter. In summer use ointment of sandal, camphor etc., which is cooling. In rainy season use sandal, saffron and musk ointment which is neither hot nor cold. Pray to the deity and give charity. In the hair musk paste be smeared.

Flowers

Wear fragrant flowers on head. It removes foul smell of sweating, stickiness and exertion. And it promotes eyesight, alleviates burning sensation and gives happiness. Wear soft petals of ketaki. With musk, wear jati pushpa, vakula, champaka, srikhanda etc. With camphor wear mandara, nilotpala, kumuda, raktotpala etc. Without bath wear mallika. After bath wear jati and bilva. During massage wear ketaki. All these flowers are similar in taste and potency. They alleviate all three humours; so they can be worn at all time. In winter wear ketaki, vakula, srikhanda, satapatra and champaka as they are hot. In rainy season, srivaka, nilotpala and srikhanda can be used as they are neither too hot nor too cold. They cure eye diseases.

Wear jati flower 18 hours, naivali 1 hour 36 minutes, utpala 3 nights, ketaki 5 nights, satapatra 3 nights, mallika half-night, champaka one day and night, yutika 1 hour 36 minutes, srikhanda, vakula and mandara one night each, sriparna only during the food.

Jati pushpa alleviates all the 3 humours and cures serious burning sensation. Utpala alleviates bile, causes non-sliminess and promotes eyesight. Ketaki alleviates mucus and wind, hot in potency, free from dust and best among flowers. Satapatra is slightly hot and fragrant and promotes eyesight. It also cures giddiness in the head.

Mallika is not good for eyes, so avoid it. Champaka alleviates wind and promotes eyesight, cures non-sliminess and auspicious. Patala is exceedingly cooling and aggravates mucus and wind, but it cures loss of power of digestion, diseases of bile and ear diseases. It also cures fever, fainting and morbid thirst. It promotes longevity and cures burning sensation.

In winter satapatra is useful; in spring ketaki, in summer naivali and malati, and in rainy season patala, and in autumn champaka.

Ornaments

Gold produces purity; auspicious and satisfaction. Gold ornaments studded with gems and jewels counteract the effects of evil position of planets.

Ten sinful acts

1. Violence, 2. Stealing, 3. Desire of unnatural things, 4. Back-biting, 5. Using strong and bad words, 6. While

quarrelling telling lies, 7. Inconsistency in word and deed, 8. Desire to enjoy others' achievements, 9. Thinking ill of others, 10. Thinking of taking away others' wealth.

Look at all creatures including ants like Himself. Don't indulge in sex before 16 years of age and after 70 years. If it is disobeyed, it results in diminution of strength.

One who eats only twice a day, passes urine 6 times a day, stools 3 times a day (2 times better), performs less of (limited) sexual acts with his own wife only or sleeps with his wife only at night (daytime in summer), lives one hundred years.

Examination of strength

What is strength? The excellent essence of tissue elements beginning from chyle and plasma and ending in semen in common (sperm in male, ovum in female) is called ojas (essence of all seven categories of tissue elements). This ojas is strength in the context of medical science. Because of the strength, the muscle tissues become stable and nourished. One remains undeterred in all efforts having excellence of voice and complexion and his/her external and internal senses are capable of performing their activities with full ability.

What is tejas (essence)? Essence is originated from fire. During gradual process of metabolism of tissue elements a substance Vasa is produced out of the fat accumulated in the abdomen. It is in excess in woman. That is tejas (essence); because of this there is softness, less soft hair, exhilaration, eyesight, stability, power of digestion and metabolism, beauty and grace in woman.

What is ojas? Ojas is the nature of water. It is unctuous, white, cold, stable, fluid, remains separate from others and soft. It is located in the heart and it is one of the excellent sustainers of life. The body along with its limbs is pervaded by this ojas.

Ojas is the essence of all seven tissue elements collected by enzymes. It dwells in the heart and is predominantly white and slightly reddish as well as yellowish and is known as ojas in the body. When the ojas is destroyed he/she succumbs to death.

Ojas has ten attributes: 1. Heaviness, 2. Coldness, 3. Softness, 4. Unctuousness, 5. Thickness, 6. Sweetness, 7. Stability, 8. Freshness, 9. Whiteness, 10. Sliminess.

The universe has two attributes — heating and cooling. So ojas is also of two types — white and yellowish red. The reduction of white in ojas leads to extreme, serious and painful conditions. If the red ojas is reduced in quantity, the body becomes full of water and the patient succumbs to instantaneous death.

Mucus in its natural state promotes strength in the form of ojas. When it is morbid, it takes the form of excreta and causes miseries. Anyhow ojas and mucus are different.

Three types of strength are: superior, inferior and moderate. Another three divisions of strength are: 1. Hereditary, 2. Gained during different stages, 3. Gained as a result of drugs and diet.

Health and body

Free from diseases, low aging process, skill in profession, proficient in spirit and scientific knowledge, clean, having compact body with all this is healthy.

One who has properly apportioned and properly separated bones, well knit and sturdy joints, well formed muscles and strong body is called compact.

If anyone faints, dies or succumbs to diseases while witnessing serious bleeding or facing serious grief or fearful situation he is very weak mentally and physically though possessed of a big physique.

Looseness and prostration of the body, vitiation of humours, exertion and inability to perform work are the signs of Visramsana—derangement of ojas (strength).

Heaviness, numbness, feeling as if covered with a wet cloth, discoloration, drowsiness, more sleep and oedema of the body caused by wind are the symptoms of Vyapta—derangement of ojas.

Fainting, wasting of muscles, stupor, delirium, unconsciousness and even death are the signs of Kshaya—derangement of strength.

1. Unctuous and hot things are wholesome for early winter.
2. Pungent, bitter and ununctuous things are wholesome for late winter.
3. Pleasing, cooling and sweet things are wholesome for summer.
4. Thin gruel and purgation are wholesome for fever.
5. Fomentation is wholesome for vomiting.
6. Inhalation and smoking are wholesome for chronic cold.

Very limited quantity of alcohol cures alcoholism. A sesame seed size of poison works like ambrosia. Equal quantity of honey and ghee are taken together, it works as a poison in the body.

Alkalis and sour make sweetness

Arecanut and betel leaf with very little lime help in manifestation of good smell, colour and taste.

Jaggery causes suppression of digestive power, but with abhaya cures it. Roasted cornflower aggravates wind which is ununctuous; but adding water drink, it is nourishing but does not aggravate wind. Dry ginger is lighter than raw ginger because of processing. Red rice is lighter than fried and ground rice. Wheat paste is heavier than wheat.

Curd (yoghurt), milk and sweets are wholesome in specific localities. Milk is wholesome in east India. Fish is wholesome in Sindhu. Oil, sour things, rhizomes and roots are wholesome in Malva and Konkan. In the north thin and thick gruel are wholesome. Wheat is wholesome in Avanti.

To some people curd (yoghurt), milk and alcohol are wholesome. To some others thin gruel, vegetable soup, cereals and wheat are wholesome.

Wholesome things produce strength instantaneously. They do not vitiate humours in excess. Generally, milk is laxative; but to some it may cause constipation.

Milk is sweet and cooling, but curd (yoghurt) has opposite qualities. Ghee is like curd (yoghurt). Buttermilk (astringent and sour) is constipative; but more sour buttermilk is laxative. Tender radish alleviates humours, but overmatured radish aggravates all of them like rhizomes.

Emetic is prescribed to cure vomiting, heart disease and phantom tumour. Enema is normally contraindication for piles and obstinate skin diseases. But in certain conditions they are useful to these diseases also.

The nature of season and humour make fever easily curable. The impurity of tissue elements makes obstinate urinary disorders and diabetes. For a patient wholesome food becomes harmful in dry form; but it is useful for obstinate urinary disorders and diabetes.

Chapter 4

MATERNITY AND PEDIATRICS

Ear—sound, eye—vision, tongue—taste, nose—smell, skin—touch, tongue—speech. Hands give things to others (donate), legs—walk, anus—elimination of waste product, genital—to urinate and for sexual enjoyment. Semen (sperm and ovum) is the output of the conglomeration of the attributes of the six tastes combined together.

Stool, urine and sweat are waste products.

There are four categories of food: chewable, eatable, lickable and drinkable.

Food that nourishes tissue elements, dhatu, ojas, strength, complexion etc., does so by the help of fire. Rejuvenation does not take place by undigested food products.

Inside the umbilicus there is a circle of moon in which there is a circle of sun. In human beings in the circle of sun, fire is present in the shape of a lamp which helps to digest the food. The lamp of fire is covered which helps to digest the food. The lamp of fire is covered with a shell of glass as embryo is covered with amniotic membrane. The fire located in the umbilicus helps to digest the food by the help of its rays. In the human body there are thirteen categories of fire: 7 each of tissue elements, 5 big elements (each has its own) and 13th is Jatharagni (digestive fire).

Digestive fire has no separate existence from bile. Bile is permeated with the attributes of fire, and it causes burning, digestion etc. When the attributes of fire are reduced in the bile, similar substances are administered for increasing it.

Clarified butter alleviates bile, but stimulates fire. Goat's milk, fish etc., which increase the quantity of bile, do not stimulate fire.

Because of anger, grief and exhaustion the heat of the body goes to the head and being associated with bile it causes grey hair, as a result of which premature greying of hair is caused.

The attributes of bile and fire are different. Bile is liquid, unctuous and moves downward and fire has opposite qualities.

Bile is not treated as different from fire, because bile has attributes like taste, potency etc., and through its treatment, fire, which has no such attributes, can be corrected. Otherwise the treatment of erratic fire which has no attributes like taste etc., is impossible. So bile is fully pervaded by fire and it is the heat of bile which is powerful, along with the bile. Fire moves in the lower abdomen and through all the openings or channels of circulation. It is called bodily fire, known as proper substratum of life and invariable dependent of the body.

The body is composed of five big elements, the diet is also of the same five elements. The diet after digestion is divided into five groups to nourish the respective attributes of the body.

Before digestion of food mucus is produced, during digestion bile and after digestion wind is produced. So the residue of the food which is without any essence is eliminated.

Food taken in appropriate time is taken to gastro-intestinal tract by the help of Prana (elan vital wind). It gets integrated by the liquid secretions and becomes soft by unctuous secretions which are produced by the stimulation of Samana wind. Food gets digested on the analogy of the cooking of rice mixed with water and placed in a vessel on the external fire. In the beginning of digestion the food consisting of 6 tastes become sweet and thus produces mucus. In the second stage because of the burning it becomes sour and during this process when the food leaves the stomach, bile is produced. After it has left stomach the watery portion from the residue gets absorbed by the process of digestion and it takes the shape of formed solid mass. During this process pungent gas is produced. Then earthy fire, watery fire, fiery fire, windy fire and ethery fire digest the five groups of attributes of food. These attributes after metabolic transformation of their material nature separately nourish those of the tissue elements. The earthy attribute of food nourishes earthy attribute of tissue elements.

By implication apart from the attributes like heaviness etc., of the drugs, these fires help in the metabolic transformation of the attributes of the big elements like water, etc., in the body.

Aphrodisiac drugs like milk etc. help in the ejaculation of semen by virtue of the excellence of their own attributes.

The seven tissue elements are: Rasa (plasma and other liquid elements of the body), Mamsa (muscle tissue), Medha (fat tissue), Asthi (bone tissue), Majja (bone marrow), Sukra (semen or sperm and ovum).

Functions of the seven tissue elements: Nourishment, life, coverage, oleation, formation of basic matrix (dharma), filling up, and procreation.

After digestion stool and urine come out as excreta, and the essence of food and drink is transformed as chyle, plasma etc. By the action of the tissue elemental fire its excreta (mucus) comes out, and the gross part remains in the matrix of plasma; and the subtle part of it is transformed into hemoglobin fraction of blood. When blood is acted upon blood tissue fire, its excreta comes out as bile, the gross part remains in the matrix of blood and the subtle part of it is transformed into muscle tissue. Its waste product comes out in the form of excreta from mouth, nose, ears, eyes and genital. Similarly the subtle part is transformed into fat tissue. Its excreta comes out as sweat, and the subtle part of medha (fat tissue) is transformed into bone tissue. Its excreta comes out as nail, big hair, small hair and beard. The subtle part of bone tissue is transformed into bone marrow. The excreta of bone marrow comes out as fatty substance in the ear, stool etc. The subtle part of the bone marrow is transformed into sperm and ovum. It does not result in the production of any excreta. Its gross part remains as sperm and ovum.

The excreta of six Dhatus are: mucus, bile, stool, urine, sweat, nail, hair, excreta of the ear and eyes and stool. Some think that beard is the excreta of sperm. Pimples of the face of young boys and girls are due to the heat of semen (sperm and ovum). So it is said that pimples on the face are the excreta of semen.

Ladies due to some reason may have less hair, but in them baldness does not appear, as they are very tender and their waste products come out from menstrual secretion and as they do not indulge in exercise they are free from baldness. Because of menstrual secretion their body becomes clean; hence no baldness.

Both blood and menstrual blood are produced from out of Rasa, but there is difference. Menstrual blood including ovum has heating nature and semen including sperm has cooling nature. Embryo is formed by their combination. So the nature of embryo is both heating and cooling.

Menstrual blood has invariably heating property. Ordinary blood has both hot and cold, sweet, unctuous, red, heavy and foul smell. Like bile it causes burning sensation.

The blood that flows during menstrual period gets accumulated in the uterus and due to wind flows through the genital tract for four days every month. After the flow a portion of it remains in the body and gets purified by the contact of the semen.

Four categories of food properly digested become semen in a month's time. The same happens about ovum in women.

During the intercourse with man, woman also ejaculates semen, but the semen of woman does not take part in conception.

The menstrual blood has foul smell and it is black. The menstruation generally starts after 14 years of age till the age of 50.

As there is no blood in the dead body, blood is also called life. Because of attachment, determination and pleasant mood, semen gets excited leading to its

Frequency of sexual reproduction in a month

Age group year	Min	Max	Seasons				Humours		
			Spring	Summer	Autumn	Winter	Vata (Wind)	Pitta (Bile)	Kapha (Mucus)
20-25	20	25	25	18	21	22	18	21	25
26-30	15	20	20	14	16	18	12	15	20
31-40	10	15	15	9	11	13	8	12	15
41-50	6	10	10	4	6	8	3	6	10
51-60	1	5	5	1	2	3	1	3	5
61-100	0-1	1-2	1-2	0-1	0-1	1-2	0-1	0-1	1-2

Excess ejaculation causes fearsome diseases.

After marriage at the age of 20-25 years

Period after Marriage	Frequency per month	
	Minimum	Maximum
up to 3 months	20	25
3 months to 1 year	15	20
1 year to 10 years	10	15
10 years to 20 years	5	15
20 years to 30 years	1	5
30 years to 70 years	0-1	1-2

Excess intercourse causes fearsome diseases.

elimination through the junction between the opening of the seminal vesicle and the urinary tract.

At a distance of half an inch towards the right side below the opening of urinary bladder, in the urinary tract the semen of man gets ejaculated.

The semen has four categories of attributes: 1. Density, heaviness, stability and honey-like smell are the attributes of earth. 2. Sweetness, liquidity, unctuousness and softness are the attributes of water. 3. Hotness of semen is fire attribute. This heat is imparted to semen by bodily fire. 4. The ejaculation of semen takes place because of the attributes of wind element. Hence semen has four limbs.

The substances having pungent and sour Vipakas reduce semen. Astringent, pungent, saline and sour tastes also reduce semen. If it is so, how semen could be a product of six tastes? Habitual intake of all tastes causes nourishment of tissue elements and it is wholesome. Such effect is not achieved by the habitual intake of only one taste. Hence the semen is the product of six tastes.

When sperm and ovum unite, the all-pervading soul along with its parts and subparts and five Pranas (elan vital) or subtle big elements gets located there by virtue of its own nature.

The universal soul who has synonyms like knower of body, producer of sensation, perceiver of the sense of touch and sense of smell, observer, taster, creator, mover, sustainer, speaker etc., by providential cause gets united with the individual soul which latter is Akshaya (which does not undergo diminution), which is non-expendable, and which is unthinkable. This union endowed with the attributes of satwa (bright), raja (dim) and tama (dark) and the characteristic features of the gods, demons and similar other objects, gets carried by wind element to enter and stay inside the womb.

When the embryo is formed, because of the subtility in the beginning the appearance is not distinctly recognizable.

For conception, husband should have the diet of clarified butter, rice, milk, sugar and sweets made of milk for one month observing celibacy. These wholesome regimens should specially be adopted by the wife also. They can have cohabitation with a view to procreating offspring. In the alternative, they should be given food consisting of sesame oil etc., which aggravate bile. By adopting these regimens the wife's menstrual blood flows for three days and she delivers the baby without any complication or pain.

During menstruation, avoid routine household work for three days, having one meal a day without meat or fish, but with more milk and milk preparations. She should sleep on separate bed during menstruation and never have sexual intercourse, as it has many harmful effects. Coitus during these days never results in conception.

Fertile lady (during menstruation) shows following characteristic features. Her face becomes plump with the expression of happiness. She feels stickiness in her mouth and teeth. She likes men's association. She talks sweetly, she feels looseness in her lower abdomen, eyes and hairs of her head. She feels twitching sensation in her upper limbs, breasts, hips, umbilicus, thighs, calf region and buttocks. She also feels excitement and anxiety.

The uterus (genital tract) becomes closed after the expiry of fertility (menstruation) period.

Cohabitation days for offspring

On the fourth day of the onset of menstruation she should take bath well and wearing white dress first of all she should meet her husband. At night keeping his right leg first on the bed let the husband lie down on the back. Then keeping her left leg first on the bed let she also lie down touching her left leg on his right leg. Both of them should pray the Almighty before entering into cohabitation. If the cohabitation is for getting a child, the day should be very auspicious. To have a son perform cohabitation on 4th, 6th, 8th and 10th days from the date of onset of menstruation. For a daughter it should be on 5th, 7th, 9th and 11th days. Cohabitation on 13th day of the onset of menstruation is prohibited as it is harmful.

On odd days after the onset of menstruation ovum becomes more effective. So cohabitation on these days (up to 11th day) bears female offspring. On even days as the ovum becomes less in quantity or less effective cohabitation on those days certainly bears male offspring.

Position of wife during cohabitation for offspring: During cohabitation wife should not assume a prone posture on her husband's chest; neither should be in her sides, because with prone posture during cohabitation vata (wind) gets aggravated and afflicts her uterus. With her right side during cohabitation, kapha (mucus) which remains in her right side gets displaced and blocks the uterus. If pressure is put on her left side during cohabitation the ovum and sperm get burnt up due to pitta (bile). So the wife should receive seed by cohabitation while lying down on her back.

Before starting and during cohabitation both of them should pray the Almighty "Oh! Almighty! Give me (us) a brave son / a beautiful daughter. Give us a progeny." Some other mantras (Om, Jeshu, Ram, etc.) can also be chanted during cohabitation.

During cohabitation if sperm is ejaculated first the male offspring will be brave, strong and sturdy. If ovum is ejaculated first the female offspring will be beautiful, sturdy and compact.

If ejaculation of both takes place simultaneously the offspring will be eunuch.

The uterus (genital tract) is like a conch shell having three whirls. The third whirl is located in the bed of the womb. The foetus lies in the uterus with its face toward the back of the mother, head upward and limbs folded. A male foetus remains in the right side of the womb, with its body folded. Female foetus remains in the left of the womb and eunuch remains in the centre of the womb.

Characteristic features of a freshly conceived lady: 1. She feels sense of satisfaction, excellent excitement and prostration in the body and pain in the cardiac region. 2. No menstrual flow, 3. Feels weakness, fainting and vomiting without any cause, 4. Salivation, anaemic look and exhaustion without effort, 5. Small hairs appear in different parts of the body, 6. Spits more and has foul smell, 7. Nipple of the breasts becomes black, 8. Feels throbbing sensation in the uterus, 9. Feels burning sensation and heaviness in the body, 10. Several likings and 11. No elimination of semen and ovum from uterus. The embryo obstructs the channels of circulation of ovum and semen. By the blood, placenta is formed and the umbilical cord is formed by the chyle. The umbilical cord gets connected with the embryo and helps in the growth. The essence of the four types of food eaten by the mother becomes chyle which is divided into three parts — one part helps in the nourishment of the body of the mother, second part is utilized for the promotion of breast milk while from the third part the foetus gets nourishment.

When a lady conceives by providential cause the menstrual blood gets divided into three parts. One part increases the plumpness of the breasts and helps in accumulation of milk in them. The second part by its strength goes to foetus to provide nourishment and the third part provides nourishment to the pregnant lady. Hence no menstrual flow. The embryo grows inside an amniotic membrane with its face downwards.

Because of grief, fasting, intake of ununctuous food, suppression of the natural urges etc., wind gets aggravated to afflict the foetus. So she should avoid all these and she should be pleasant always.

Within a night of conception there is a jelly-like formation. Within 5 nights it becomes like bubbles. Within 10 nights it takes the shape of blood. Within a fortnight it becomes like a muscle. In two months it becomes compact and grows in five different directions, and because of the effect of the wind and fire the head, shoulders, lower limbs and upper limbs are formed. In the third month all the limbs and organs appear simultaneously, and the umbilical cord appears in the umbilicus of the foetus. With the help of umbilical cord, the foetus gets nourishment, and this cord has also connection to the thighs and lower abdomen of the body. The chyle produced out of food passes through the cord for the nourishment of the foetus and it results in the growth of the foetus. During the fourth month intellect begins to develop. During fifth month stomach, colon, urinary bladder, pelvis, kidney, liver, rectum, spleen, small intestine, and heart appear. Then the lady possesses two hearts — one of her own and the other of the foetus. During this period her desires should be fulfilled. If not, she procreates dumb, speaking indistinctly through her nose and malformed child. During the 6th month plasma vessels appear in the heart of embryo and holes appear in the ears. In the seventh month vessels, ligaments, bones, phalanges (each bone of fingers and toes), hairs on the head, small hairs, nails, and skin appear and the embryo becomes more conscious. At least by the end of this month sexual intercourse should completely be stopped. By ignorance, if it is performed, the foetus gets afflicted and miscarriage may happen. The foetus does not survive by such act of cohabitation.

The ojas migrates to the heart of the foetus, and the child becomes black, bluish black, greasy black due to metabolic transformation of tissue elements. The foetus born during this period does not survive.

During the eighth month there is instability in the ojas. If delivery takes place during this period, the child will not survive, because of the absence of ojas and also the affliction from southwest direction. So in this period sacrificial offerings, food etc. should be offered. A day after eight months or any day in ninth month or 10th month of pregnancy, normal delivery takes place without any complication.

During ninth month the foetus gets matured. During tenth month it develops hateful dispositions. It feels, staying in the mother's womb is like a hell, because of the presence of stool and urine. If it gets a chance to get out of it, it would pray the Lord, so that it would never be required to come to mother's womb again.

It is also necessary to note that the fresh pregnant lady after three months should not stay on prone posture. The cohabitation should be when she lies on her sides.

Humours located in the heart get pressed by the foetus to produce signs and symptoms of heaviness, emaciation, oedema in feet, vomiting, loss of strength and complexion, from fourth month onwards in pregnant ladies.

To alleviate itching use butter. To stop burning sensations inside the body eat sweet balls prepared with fenugreek, sesame, clarified butter and sugar. During 5th month she becomes excessively emaciated. During 6th month the foetus gets more strength and complexion than the mother. So she feels more diminution. If the mother during her bicardiac stage wears the dress and ornaments, and enjoy the food and regimens of the different countries, the child will be resembling the inhabitant of that country. If she desires a child with big eyes, strong heart and thick hairs of the head she should eat rice mixed with sesame oil and rice with soup. If she longs during her bicardiac stage to see a disciplined saint in a hermitage she delivers a religious child.

The pregnant lady should avoid: 1. Remaining awake at night, 2. Sleeping during the daytime, 3. Sitting on a hard seat, 4. Irregular postures of the body, 5. Anger, envy, worry, fear and exhaustion, 6. Fasting, intake of food in large quantity, 7. Suppression of urges, hunger, thirst, 8. Excessive cohabitation, 9. Irritating foods and drinks, 10. Suppression of desire of liking things and 11. Things which are sharp, hot, heavy and gas forming in the colon.

If she resorts to the above, it may cause abortion, emanation of foetus or its death. The table shows the characteristic features of the child according to the food and regimen of the mother's pregnancy.

No.	Food and Regimen of Mother	Characteristic features of foetus (child)
1.	Alcoholic drinks	The child will be constantly thirsty without energy.
2.	Habitual cohabitation	The child will be shameless. Life span will be short.
3.	Excessive sleep	Less power of speech, less intellect and more drowsiness.
4.	Habitual awakening at night	The child also awakes; it will be thin and weak.
5.	Constant grief	Child will be disfigured and weak, short span of life.
6.	Jealousy	Child will be of warm disposition: ferocious and envious.
7.	Ego	Child possesses more strength and inflicts miseries to others.

8.	Excess tired	Child will be quarrelsome, lazy in its own duties.
9.	Moving naked	Child will be insane.
10.	Constantly quarrelsome disposition	Child will be epileptic.
11.	Eating cold and stale food	Child may have excessive instability of mind.
12.	Habitually eating meat	Child will be asthmatic.
13.	Intake of goat meat	The child may have two heads.
14.	Habitual sweet eating	Child may suffer from diseases of mucus, fatty dump and diabetic.
15.	Habitual sour taking	Child may suffer from bleeding, eye diseases, obstinate skin disease, leprosy and erysipelas.
16.	Excess salt	Child may cause premature wrinkling, graying, and baldness.
17.	Habitual pungent taking	Child becomes weak, less semen, less eyesight, less sexual power.
18.	Habitual bitter taking	Child may have wind diseases, dry skin and less strength.
19.	Habitual astringent taking	Child may have diseases of blood and constipation.

Check the diet and regimens and correct.

Characteristic features of the lady to deliver a male offspring:

Appearance of lactation first in the right breast.

Enlargement of size of the right eye.

Prominence of right thigh.

Thinking of male offspring during bicardiac state.

Dreams of lotus flowers and mangoes.

Appearance of happiness in the face and freshness of complexion.

The characteristic features are opposite to the above indicated if the child is female.

Table showing the age of mother and sex of the expected offspring

Mon.	Age of Mother																											
	18	19	20	21	22	23	24	25	26	27	28	29	30	31	32	33	34	35	36	37	38	39	40	41	42	43	44	45
Jan	F	M	F	M	F	M	M	F	M	F	M	F	M	M	M	F	M	M	F	M	F	M	F	M	F	M	M	F
Feb	M	F	M	F	M	M	F	M	F	M	F	M	F	F	F	M	F	M	M	F	M	F	M	F	M	F	M	M
Mar	F	M	F	F	M	F	M	M	M	F	M	F	F	M	M	M	M	F	M	M	F	M	F	M	F	M	F	M
Apr	M	F	M	F	F	M	M	F	F	M	F	F	F	F	F	M	F	M	F	M	M	M	M	F	M	F	M	F
May	M	F	M	F	M	M	F	F	F	F	F	M	F	F	F	F	F	F	M	F	M	M	F	M	F	M	M	F
Jun	M	M	M	F	F	F	M	M	M	F	F	M	F	F	F	F	F	F	F	M	F	F	M	F	M	F	M	F
Jul	M	M	M	F	F	M	M	F	F	M	M	M	F	F	F	F	F	F	F	F	M	F	M	M	F	M	F	M
Aug	M	M	M	F	M	F	F	M	M	M	M	M	F	F	F	M	F	M	F	M	F	M	F	M	M	F	M	F
Sep	M	M	M	F	F	M	F	M	F	M	M	M	F	F	F	F	F	F	M	F	M	F	M	F	M	M	F	M
Oct	M	M	F	F	F	M	F	M	F	M	M	F	F	F	F	F	F	F	M	M	F	M	F	M	F	M	M	F
Nov	M	F	M	F	F	M	F	M	F	F	F	F	M	F	F	F	M	M	M	F	M	F	M	F	M	M	F	M
Dec	M	F	M	F	F	F	F	M	F	M	F	F	M	M	M	M	M	M	M	M	F	F	F	M	F	M	F	M

There may be some change if the delivery is in 8th or 9th month. Nowadays the doctors can foretell by screening after 5 months the sex of the offspring in mother's womb. So this table is not important.

There are seven layers of skin:

Avabhasini: It carries lymph and water. Padmakantaka and sidhma diseases are located here.

Lohita dhara: Tila kalaka disease is located here.

Sveta: Carma dala disease is located here.

Tamra: Kitasa and suitra diseases are located here.

Vedini: Leprosy, dadru and gaja carma are the diseases.

Mamsa dhara: Abscess, fistula in ano, piles are the main diseases.

Lohita: Diseases like galaganda, ganda mala, balmika, slipada are located here.

Besides nine external openings the tenth opening is the opening in the anterior fontanelle for male and for female three additional openings are two openings of the breasts and the genital tract through which the menstrual blood flows.

The eight kinds of joints are:

Ball and socket joint, e.g., axilla (shoulder), chest, thigh (hip) and teeth.

Mandala: Located in throat, cardiac region, eyes and trachea.

Saṃudga (two vessels kept face to face and sealed): Located in hip, shoulder, anal region and legs.

Luna Sevini: Located in head and hip.

Sankhavasta: Located in ears and sphenoidal region.

Pratora: Located in the neck and vertebral column. This joint has the shape of spear (pratara).

Kora: Located in wrist, ankle, knee and elbow. This joint has the shape of an ear or a bud (kora).

Vayasatundika: Located in the mandibular region and both the thighs.

In the human body there are 107 marmas (vital spots) which are of 5 varieties — vital spots in the muscles, vital spots having the vessels, vital spots having ligaments and nerves, vital spots in the bones and vital spots in the joints. These marmas are divided into 5 categories: 1. Which cause instantaneous death, 2. Which cause death after some time, 3. Which cause death when the foreign body is taken out, 4. Which cause deformity and 5. Which cause pain. For more details please refer to my book "Ayurvedic Massage and Healing".

Numbness of the body, heaviness, unconsciousness, desire for cold things, fainting, vomiting and dyspnoea are the signs and symptoms of a person whose vital spots are injured. If there is injury to ligaments and nerves and muscle vital spots, the signs and symptoms manifested and the treatment are described elaborately in the chapter dealing with the treatment of fresh wounds in Kharanada Samhita.

Process of death

The arteries which are made up of five big elements effect an intimate contact between the five sensory faculties and the five sensory organs for five times. Thereafter, these five sensory faculties establish contact with the five big elements at the time of the death or disintegration of five big elements of the individual.

The equilibrium of humours etc. is determined by inference. The characteristic features of equilibrium of humours in the body are:

There is regular desire for food.

Feels comfortable, when takes light food.

Proper digestion of the ingested food.

Is endowed with excellent complexion and strength.

Proper elimination of flatus, stool and urine and ejaculation of semen.

The five senses are able to perceive their objects properly.

Sleeps well.

A healthy person is he who has equilibrium of humours, fires, tissue elements, excreta and other activities of the body, who has happiness of individual soul, sense and mind.

The object of therapeutics is to prevent any change in the equilibrium of tissue elements and to maintain the continuity of tissue elements which are in a state of equilibrium.

Remedial measures be adopted for cold during winter and for hot during summer. Never ignore the time when there is indication for administration of the therapy. It should be over by the time the transformation of chyle or plasma takes place.

Chapter 5

PREDICTION BY OBSERVING THE SYMPTOMS

Messengers' role to know the result of treatment

Appearance, talk, dress and movement, 2. Location of the star, time of day and night, day of the fortnight (tithi) when the physician is called, 3. Auspicious or inauspicious events, 4. Bird's characteristic feature, wind and locality, 5. Speech, movement of the body and mental action of physician.

If the messenger is of the same caste and clan as the patient, he is auspicious and successful. Messenger wearing white cloth, hands full of presents, betel leaf in mouth, skilful, good conduct, and intelligent, all this results in happiness.

The messenger comes from north, west or northwest, peaceful, speaks smilingly to the physician, talks skilfully in moderate voice, requests the physician to grace the patient, intelligent, expert in accomplishing his own objectives — then the disease will be cured.

Meeting of messenger and physician near the dam is good for patients suffering from Rakta pitta (bleeding from several parts of the body), diarrhea, obstinate urinary disorder and diabetes.

Woman messenger is not conducive to auspiciousness. Two persons should not be sent as messenger. Such a man is not useful as a messenger who is disabled, a patient, having grief and crying.

Messenger having oil in his hand or a vehicle of donkey and the patient suffers from T.B., the physician should not go there.

Messenger of a bile patient meets the physician when the messenger is sweating or afflicted with heat, midday or near fire it is inauspicious. But it is auspicious if the patient is suffering from mucus.

The messenger of the vomiting or diarrhea patient meets the physician in a house having semen and urine is bad.

If treatment is administered on an auspicious day, the result will be good. While going to the patient, the physician's first sight (Sakunam) should be king, elephant, peacock, washerman with washed clothes, young lady with a child, prostitute or virgin girl are auspicious. Meat, water pot, umbrella, horse, elephant, unripe fruit, cow with calf, curd, gold, vessel full of unbroken rice, gem and flowers are auspicious. While going hearing the sound of swan from physician's left side, horse itches its right side, the treatment will be successful. A couple of donkeys itching each other's neck with their teeth the patient will be cured.

While entering into the patient's house if the physician sees a crying woman in his right side it is good. If the lady is passionate, it is also good. If the lady shakes her body it is not good. During journey if the physician sees a procession of a dead body without crying it is good. Cordial speech just before the onset of journey is good. While going seeing a snake on the left side is good. On seeing a snake if it raises its head endows the person with a kingdom. During journey pleasing mind of the physician is good.

When the span of life is coming to an end there will be less excessive or irregular manifestation of the natural characteristic features and graceful appearance of the person will disappear. If there is catabolic process in the tissue elements in the sensory organs which are the receptors of the senses there will be manifestation of signs and symptoms. Then the death occurs immediately.

If the patient keeps his palm flat and extends backward his middle and index fingers automatically extend his death is certain.

Frequent trembling in umbilicus, arms and palate and goat's smell comes from the body — he will not survive. Body getting cold, producing hum sound, air through mouth is hot and nose is cold — he lives 6 hours.

One looks up being afflicted with heat, lips black and thick, no sensation of touch, he survives two days.

Tongue black, face red, pain in the heart, giddiness, delusion of mind, suffers from dyspnoea, having thin voice — he lives three days.

Unable to see the tips of nose, tongue and lips which he was able to see previously — he dies on the 4th day.

If there is no horripilation by fanning and sprinkling water frequently he lives only 5 nights.

Immediately after bath heart, palms and sole get dried he lives 6 nights.

If one is unable to recognize the cold of the ice or hot things, within 8 days he dies.

If one is unable to see his head through ghee, oil, water or mirror he lives 10 nights.

If one sees other person without head or in reverse manner he dies on 12th day.

If one sees stars in daytime, sky being clear sees dust everywhere, sees lightning when there are no clouds and sees rainbow at night — he dies within 2 months.

When one's three middle fingers become suddenly curved without disease, throat dries; memory fails frequently and suddenly becomes dumb — he dies in six months.

If there is sudden increase in the size of head, drinking adequate water, still his thirst is not quenched, having enough food still he has no satisfaction — he dies in seven months.

When the sky is clear if one sees the sun as black, cold earth — he dies in 9 months.

If one's ears, hands, legs, nostrils, face, tip of penis become grayish blue — he dies in 10 months.

If the base of the thumb does not move, he is a T.B. patient and dies within a year.

If from the body or head particles like powder of cow-dung cake fall in large quantity, he is as dead.

If the fragrance of different flowers emanates from the body day and night it is the sign of imminent death.

If there are no excreta in the eyes, he succumbs to death.

The three bodies

Body	Composition	State	Existence	Gunas (Qualities)
1. Gross (Physical)	Gross element from food	Waking	Physical	Tamas
2. Subtle (Astral)	Subtle elements from impressions	Dream	Astral	Rajas
3. Casual	Casual element from Gunas (Qualities)	Deep sleep	Casual (ideal)	Satwa
Pure consci-ousness transcendent beyond self	Unmodified Consciousness	Turiya	Absolute	Nirguna

Dreams—Fruitless

1. Dreams based on things already experienced, heard, seen, requested and thought. 2. Dreams of long duration disturbed and well manifested, 3. Dreams in daytime due to aggravation of wind, 4. Dreams due to fullness of bladder (by urine), and rectum (by stool). Dreams caused by factors other than the above are fruitful dreams.

Virtuous acts bring auspicious dreams. Sinful acts bring inauspicious dreams.

When the channel of mind gets obstructed by wind etc., one gets dreams caused by different humours. By aggravation of wind one gets dreams of dances, songs, sex indulgence, movement on vehicles, fall, swimming, running and flying into the sky.

If bile is aggravated one gets dreams of quarrels, beating, anger, heat, black, red and yellow colour, sour taste and dazzling objects.

By aggravation of mucus one dreams of sleep, laziness, water, sweet taste, cold things and excessively heavy articles.

Dream in the first 3 hours of night (1st yama) produces result within one year. Dream during second 3 hours (2nd yama) produces result in 8 months and dream during third 3 hours (3rd yama) produces result in 3 months. Dream at the time of sunrise produces result within 10 days.

All white things except cotton, ash, bone, skull and root in the dream provide happiness. But cotton etc. indicate danger or disease.

All black things except cow, bird, swan and fish in dream are despicable and they take away health and fame.

Dreams of bud, flower, fruit, black bee, umbrella, flag, curd (yoghurt), cloth, food, betel, arecanut, lotus, jar, conch shell, ornaments, gold, sun, moon and stars are auspicious.

If a patient dreams of lotus flower, pond full of lotus flowers and water, hands in blessing posture, swimming in the sea, intake of milk, alcohol or blood, procurement of wealth, and happiness, he will be cured of the disease.

Drinking of milk in dream is auspicious. Drinking of alcohol, ghee, thin gruel, milk preparation etc. in dreams leads to happiness.

Dreams of heap of paddy, sesame, rice, wheat, mustard, barley etc., a creeper with flowers, tree with fruits and procurement of wealth indicate recovery from the disease.

In the dream if one embraces a beautiful lady wearing white dress it is the sign of happiness.

By dreaming of snake, scorpion etc., one does not get terrified; he acquires wealth.

If a lady dreams of the incision of her genital organ she gets her husband. If she dreams of fruits she gets wealth. If she dreams of dazzling objects she regains her health. If she dreams of menstruation she gains happiness.

If one dreams of an empty house or temple without idol, fall of tree having flowers, honey, oil, oil cake, metals, salt, sesame seed, boiled rice, drinking wine, taking bath, animals with ferocious face smell him frequently etc., he succumbs to death.

If in dream, one climbs a tree full of flowers — his death is not far off.

If one dreams of taking water he dies of diabetes or diarrhea.

If one dreams of being fanned by lotus he dies of leprosy. If one dreams of growth of tree in his abdomen he dies of phantom tumour. If one dreams of growth of tree in his head he dies of headache. If one dreams of eating he dies of vomiting. If one dreams of taking honey he dies of asthma and morbid thirst. If one dreams of eating turmeric he dies of anaemia. If one dreams of taking blood he dies of bleeding from several parts of the body (Rakta pitta). If one dreams of vomiting rice with meat facing the south he dies of wind diseases. If one dreams of vomiting grapes and other sour things he dies of bile diseases. If one dreams of vomiting or a dwarf he dies of mucus diseases.

If one dreams of singing and dancing by climbing a palace of gold or enters into a dark cave, sinks into a dark well, enters into crematorium or flood water, receiving gold, witnessing the cracking of mountain, he succumbs to death.

If one dreams of a lady in red or black dress, her hair loose, having big hands, crying, singing, chewing her teeth, dragging, hugging, kissing and calling with wrath and anger at night he succumbs to death. One, having such dreams, should recite Mrityunjaya and Gayatri mantras. Never speak of his evil dreams to others. Let him reside in a temple or auspicious place for three nights.

Three forms of Lord Vishnu (Rama, Krishna, Govinda), three channels of Ganga (Ganga, Yamuna, Saraswati), three eyes of Rudra (Rudra, Siva, Sankara) — remembering all these counteract the effects of bad dreams.

Chapter 6

DIAGNOSIS

EXAMINING THE PATIENT

Ayurveda does not consider the pulse as mere cardiovascular index. It represents the physiological and pathological condition of entire body. The expert pulse readers claim that the perfect knowledge of pulse can help in diagnosis of the diseases and also impending death of the patient.

Pulse examination

Examine the pulse early morning when the stomach is empty. It is prohibited to examine the pulse immediately after bath, food and oil massage; as the pulse becomes erratic and does not indicate correct condition. Don't examine the pulse when the patient is hungry and thirsty.

The radical artery pulse is about half an inch below the thumb. Examine the pulse of males on the right and females on the left. The hand should be in slightly flexed position. The physician examines the pulse using index, middle and ring fingers of his right hand; keeping the index finger near the thumb of the patient. Uniform pressure is applied through the fingertips on the pulse. See which finger feels strong pulsation. If the strong pulsation is on the tip of the index finger, wind is dominant, middle indicates pitta (bile) and ring indicates aggravation of mucus. Observe the movement of pulse. If the motion is like a snake or leech, it indicates wind, motion of crow, sparrow or frog indicates bile, and the motion of swan, peacock or cock indicates mucus. If the motion is like snake and sometimes frog, it is the sign of aggravation of both wind and bile. The motion of snake and swan indicates the aggravation of wind and mucus. If the movement is like frog and swan, it indicates both bile and mucus are aggravated. When all three humours are vitiated the pulse moves like woodpecker bird. Elaborate examination of pulse in different diseases is made by the physician as the means to probe the diseases.

If the pulsation is in the same manner in its own place for at least 30 times, the patient survives. If not, he does not survive more. If the pulsation is after pauses it indicates impending death. If the pulsation is in a curved manner, in a sluggish manner, irregular manner after pauses and if the pulsation is very thin, he succumbs to death. If the pulsation is felt in the sides of the shoulder and then in the fingertips it is the pulse of sannipata which is incurable. If the pulse bears the characteristic of bile in the beginning, then wind and mucus respectively, if it shifts from its place very frequently, if it moves like a wheel, if it beats fiercefully after pauses and if it is thready, the patient does not recover. Thick beating indicates that the pulse carries nutrients of muscle tissue. During fever the pulse is hot having a faster beat. During passion and anger the pulse beats faster. During worry and fear it is thready. If the digestive fire is weak and suffers diminution of tissue element, the pulse becomes very subtle. If the pulse is full of blood, it is warm. If there is ama the pulse will be heavy. If the digestive fire is strong the pulse will be light but beats fast. If the patient is hungry there is instability in pulsation. After satisfaction of food the pulse becomes stable. If the pulsation is very fast and if it is covered with excreta the patient will have high fever within half a day. During death pulsation is like old damaru (a kind of pan). He may survive for a day. When the heart, nose, hands and feet become cold, his pulsation is fast but subtle, he dies soon.

Tibetan pulse examination

The arteries of the patient are like messengers between the doctor and the patient. There are some general rules for the doctor and the patient before pulse examination.

For the patient: Previous evening should have light diet, exertion or sitting in the hot sun is prohibited; but should rest well, to avoid the disturbances of bile and wind to make a clear diagnosis.

For the doctor: The doctor must be well prepared and relaxed before examination, to obtain good result. The pulse is examined just an inch from the wrist as it is the closest to the vital organs of the body. Pulsating the vein on the leg is unsuitable as it is far from the vital organs. For examination, index, middle and ring fingers are used which should be held in a line close to one another but not touching each other. More pressure should be applied by the middle finger and ring finger.

Examine the patient's left hand by doctor's right. (a) The tip of the index finger on the right side detects heart diseases; on the left intestinal diseases. (b) The tip of the middle finger on the right detects diseases affecting the spleen and on the left stomach diseases. (c) The tip of the ring finger on the right detects kidney diseases and on the left diseases affecting the seminal vesicle.

Examine the patient's right hand by doctor's left. (a) Right tip of the index detects lung diseases, the left tip diseases of the guts. (b) Right tip of the middle finger detects liver, left tip detects unbalanced bile. (c) Right tip of the ring finger detects kidney, left tip diseases of urinary bladder.

Examine the female's right hand first, and left hand first of the male, because the tip of the female heart is tilted towards the right and vice versa with male.

Chinese pulse examination

Chinese think that the pulsation is the indication of perfection of the art of medicine. Pulse examination does not only give the present state of health, but tells also of the diseases of the past and predicts the diseases that may appear in future. Right and left wrist pulses are examined, putting three fingers and with each finger the pulse is felt in the segment under that finger by light and deep touch respectively. Thus total 12 observations including both sides.

The best time for pulse test is about 3 a.m., when the stomach is empty. The distal deep pulse felt at left is heart, the middle deep is liver and the proximal deep is kidney. Superficial pulses respectively are small intestine, gall bladder, and urinary bladder respectively. On the right deep in the same order are lung, spleen and circulation, sex, and superficially the large intestine, stomach and triple wormer. The pulses identify the organs diseased and so the meridians affected. The meridians give the most effective acupressure point to relieve pain and suffering.

Urine test (Ayurveda)

Though there is no systematic description of urine test in Ayurvedic classics, its characteristic features in different diseases are described. Urine is collected just before dawn. Leave the first flow, the middle flow urine is collected in a clean glass which should be covered with a clean cloth preventing it from dust and flies. After the sun rises bring it to the light and stir it well and observe whether there is obstinate disorders including diabetes, colour and its Nirama and Sama conditions.

Put a drop of oil on the surface of the urine. If the oil spreads instantaneously the disease is curable. If not, difficult to cure. If the oil goes down to settle at the bottom of the container, the disease is incurable. After dropping oil through a straw, if bubbles appear it indicates that the disease is of bile. If the disease is of wind, the urine is unctuous and looks like waste product muscle fat. The oil drop remains stagnant on the surface of the urine. If mucus is aggravated, the urine appears like muddy tank water. Due to aggravation of wind, the urine becomes blue, transparent, unctuous, cold and black. Due to bile aggravation, it becomes reddish and oily. By mucus aggravation, it becomes unctuous, thick like muddy tank water. By vitiation of blood, the urine becomes unctuous, hot, red and thick. Due to indigestion the urine looks like the juice of vinegar, simple water or sandalwood paste. Due to aggravation of wind in its Nirama the urine becomes transparent and white. If the urine is like rice wash and smells like the urine of a goat or a donkey, it is the sign of indigestion. By increasing Rasa dhatu the urine will be like sugarcane juice, netlike or reddish. Then fasting is good. During the first stage of fever the urine is of smoky colour with profuse urination.

When bile and wind are aggravated, the urine is like slight hot smoke water.

If wind and mucus are aggravated, the urine will be white with bubbles.

When mucus and bile are aggravated the urine is of cloudy red colour.

If the urine is like blood and yellow, he suffers from chronic fever.

During sânnipata (simultaneous vitiation of all three humours) the urine is black but transparent.

If the urine is black with yellow at the bottom the patient suffers from Amavata (rheumatism) and vitiation of mucus.

During Nirama fever, the urine is yellow or red and foamy. During head disease the urine appears like the water of umbrella with foam.

If the urination is after a long time with ununctuous yellow and white, it indicates mild disease and gets cured by wholesome diet.

The gout (Rakta Vata) patient's urine is black with bubbles as well as netlike substance in it.

Obstinate skin disease patient's urine is like the urine of horse. Due to aggravation of wind in the upper part of the body, the lower urine is white and the upper urine is blue and unctuous.

In the case of patients of blood diarrhea or vomiting or facial paralysis, the lower portion of the urine is like either buttermilk or oil and upper urine is red.

Simple diarrhea patient's urine is redder at the bottom.

If the urine is yellow or like the urine of a dog and the patient feels laziness, it is the sign of jaundice. It can be cured easily.

If the patient urinates in small quantity having black or red colour he has infestation by intestinal worms.

If the patient has heart pain the urine is like donkey's. When there is simultaneous aggravation of all the three humours, the urine is yellow or blue with bubbles.

If the oil drop over the urine spreads and the urine is black he is a T.B. patient. If the urine is white it is incurable.

The urine of the patient of obstinate abdominal diseases including ascites is like meat-wash.

If the urination is with difficulty and if the lower urine is yellow, he has rheumatism and vitiation of mucus.

If the patient passes urine white above and yellow below, and if the urine looks like water below and yellow above with bubbles, he suffers from burning syndrome of hands and feet. It can be cured.

The urine of the patient having pain in eyes is like donkey's urine, colour yellow with bubbles. If there is association of obstinate abdominal diseases including ascites the urine becomes blue.

The urine of the patient having tongue and teeth diseases is white with red bubbles.

In ascites the urine becomes like drops of clarified butter. The urine of the patient of stony inflammation of parotid gland looks netted as saffron.

The urine of the patient having postpartum infection is yellowish with black bubbles.

If original water-like urine instantaneously changes to oil colour on keeping in a pot, the patient succumbs to death.

On dropping oil over the urine if it suddenly spreads to the east the patient recovers soon. If oil spreads to south he has fever and slowly recovers. If oil spreads to north he certainly recovers. If the oil spreads to northeast, he dies within a month. If the oil spreads to southeast or southwest and if holes appear in it he certainly dies. If the oil spreads northwest he dies though he has taken ambrosia. If the oil spreads to west he recovers and gets happiness.

If the oil drop sometimes floats, sometimes sinks and sometimes moves in the urine of a moribund patient, he never survives.

If the oil drop takes the shape of plough, tortoise, circle, man without head, conch shell, sword, pastel and mortar, arrow, stick, crossing of three or four roads, or drop, don't treat the patient.

If the oil drop takes the shape of swan, lotus, elephant, tail of yak, umbrella, gate or a palatial building in complete form, by treatment he surely recovers.

If the oil drop takes the shape of triangle he is afflicted by fault of clan.

If the drop of oil takes the shape of human being or two heads, he suffers from affliction of evil spirit. Necessary steps should be taken to correct the evil spirit.

If the stream of micturition is white or yellowish, he suffers from acute fever. If the stream is red, he is overcome by a chronic disease. If the stream is black he succumbs to death.

Mala (stool) test

There are 16 types of morbidities in stool. 1. Foul smell in excess, 2. No smell or having different type of smell, 3. Bluish gray, 4. Broken pieces of stool, 5. White,

6. Reddish, 7. Brown or black, 8. Cold to touch, 9. Looseness, 10. Foams, 11. Greenish, 12. Scybalous stool, 13. Smoky, 14. Several colours, 15. Black, 16. Stool which is both compact and loose.

Broken and foamy stool indicates several vata (wind). Green or yellow stool is the sign of aggravated pitta (bile). Horripilation and excess stool in white colour, and feeling cold by touch and more compact is the sign of aggravation of mucus.

Bluish black and white stool denotes the disease of wind and mucus. More foul smell and loose stool is due to stool accumulation in colon since long time. Yellowish, compact but in pieces is due to wind-bile. Stool afflicted by ama and wind with yellowishness is the sign of bile.

When the child passes stool blue-black, foamy, spreading on the floor, having less temperature in the body, take the child to the doctor. Broken, bluish black stool denotes aggravation of wind. Yellow and blue stool is of bile and white stool indicates mucus. White stool with more foul smell is the sign of starting of ascites. Bluish black stool denotes constipation.

Black or bluish black with most foul smell stool, or hot stool with the smell of dead body indicates his death.

Eye test

If the eyes are dry, smoky and fierceful, if the eyeball is mobile and if there is burning sensation, there is aggravation of bile.

During mucus aggravation, there will be watering of the eyes, anxious look, no gaze in the eyes, the eyeballs move and the eyesight will be weak.

If one eye is fierceful and the other is closed, he dies within 3 days.

If the black of the eye (iris) loses its glaze, if the eyeballs go inside and if the vision is bluish black the patient certainly dies.

If the eyes are red or black and if the look is fierceful the patient certainly dies.

If there is fixed look, if he is unconscious with delirium and cracks in the pupil, he dies within a day.

Tongue test

Elan vital moves through the tongue. It is the most important among the subtle senses. By examination of tongue four conditions could be ascertained:

Whether he has fever or has come free from it.

Aggravation of wind, bile and mucus separately.
Aggravation of all the three humours simultaneously.

Curable or incurable.

Due to aggravation of wind, the tongue will be like leaf having numbness and cracks.

If bile is aggravated, the tongue is red with burning sensation and it will be covered with thorn-like growth.

By aggravation of mucus the tongue is heavy, thick, excessively cold, white and thickly coated.

When all 3 humours are simultaneously aggravated the tongue is ununctuous, bitter, as if burnt, rough touch and having deep cracks.

Teeth examination

The morbidity of teeth is of seven types: brown, red, black, reddish, yellow, having bleeding and retraction of the gum from the roots of teeth.

Due to aggravation of wind teeth become blue. So measures for alleviation of it should be adopted. Because of aggravation of bile, teeth become brown, so alleviate bile.

On mucus aggravation teeth become red with other characteristic features. Black teeth is the aggravation of wind and bile. Bluish brown teeth is due to other features. One who has stomatitis has reddish teeth. When there is simultaneous aggravation of wind and mucus he suffers from inflammation and glossitis.

In diseases of bile and mucus there will be exudation from teeth and nose.

Adhesion of excreta in the root of teeth is the premonitory sign of obstinate urinary diseases and diabetes.

Nail examination

Due to aggravation of wind the nails become blue. If the nails are red or yellow it indicates aggravation of bile. If the nails are white, mucus is aggravated. On simultaneous aggravation of wind and bile, the nails become bluish yellow or bluish red.

If nails are either yellow or red, it denotes the aggravation of mucus and bile.

When all three humours are simultaneously aggravated, if the colour of the nails becomes reddish blue, yellow, green, white and free from dirt the patient dies.

Prediction of the death date

With the help of the preceptor attain perfection in the mantra, "KAPALA RUDRAYA BHAGAVATE NAMAH". Let the person in his own blood write it over the leaf of burja and keep it inside two earthen plates in a secret place. After oblation recite the mantra repeatedly. In the morning get up from the bed, open the container and examine the mantra. If any alphabet has become invisible count the number of remaining alphabet. Death will occur in the same number of year or month or day.

Another method of prediction: In three columns names of twenty-seven stars beginning from Ardra and ending with Margasira in the order shown below having Mula in the centre:

6. Ārdrā	7. Punarvasu	8. Puṣyā
11. Pūrva Phālguni	10. Magha	9. Aslesā
12. Uttara Phālguni	13. Hastā	14. Citrā
17. Anurādhā	16. Viśākhā	15. Swati
18. Jyesthā	19. Mula	20. Purva Āśādhā
23. Dhanisthā	22. Sravaṇa	21. Uttarāṣādhā
24. Śatabhisā	25. Pūrva Bhadrapada	26. Uttara Bhadrapada
2. Bharani	1. Asvini	27. Revati
3. Krittika	4. Rohini	5. Margaśirā

If the moon, sun and the star of the time of birth remain in one column the patient succumbs to death, otherwise he survives.

To know the nature of death time for himself or for others, the physician observing celibacy fasts on 11th day of bright fortnight (Sukla Ekadasi) of the month Margasirsa. After offering prayer with purity of mind he writes over a wooden plate with sandalpaste water the twelve-alphabet mantra, "Om Namo Bhagavate Vasudevaya". Offering prayer to Hari and with purity the wise man looks at it for one year.

If the first letter is invisible the patient dies in 3 hours on Thursday of Margasirsa.

If the second letter is invisible the patient with fever dies in the evening of Monday on 5th day of bright fortnight in the month of Pausha.

If the 3rd letter is invisible the patient afflicted by evil planets and fever dies in the afternoon of Sunday of full moon or new moon.

If the 4th letter is invisible the patient with fever dies on Friday noon, 9th day of bright fortnight in the month of Phalguna.

If 5th letter is invisible the patient with diarrhea dies early morning of Tuesday in the month of Caitra.

If 6th letter is invisible the patient dies at night of Thursday on 13th day of the fortnight in the month of Vaisakha.

If 7th letter is invisible the patient having oedema and constipation dies at night after 3 hours in the month of Jyestha.

If 8th letter is invisible the patient with diarrhea dies at noon Sunday on 8th day of black fortnight in Asadha.

If 9th letter is invisible the patient dies in the first part of night of the month of Asadha or Sravana.

If 10th letter is invisible he dies by snakebite at night of Sunday on 12th day of bright fortnight of the month of Bhadrapada.

If 11th letter is invisible the patient with fever and ascites (obstinate abdominal diseases) dies in the afternoon of 8th day of black fortnight of Asvina.

If the 12th letter is invisible the patient with diarrhea dies on 5th day of bright fortnight of Kartika month.

If the relatives and friends of the patient will be extremely grieved by disclosing the patient's death, the physician should not disclose it and should not treat the patient also.

Towards a moribund patient several evil spirits are daily attracted. They counteract the potency of drugs, because of their desire to kill the patient. So most effective therapy also fails to produce good result.

If a physician has to treat an incurable patient, having bad prognostic signs and symptoms, he should advise the patient to visit religious places and offer charity. Without that by mere treatment the disease cannot be cured. Only Vishnu can alleviate such diseases.

To overcome such situations let the patient recite Mrityunjaya mantram, Vishnu Sahasranamam, and Mahakala mantram.

Chapter 7

ABOUT THE BODY (ACCORDING TO MODERN SCIENCE)

ANATOMY AND PHYSIOLOGY

The study of the structure of the body is Anatomy and Physiology is the study of the functions of the parts of the body. Gross anatomy is the study without the help of microscope. Regional, embryological, systemic, developmental and radiographic are the subdivisions of anatomy which can be studied with the help of microscope. Hence it is called microscopic anatomy.

Atom to organism

The body is composed of atoms, the basic unit of all matter. When two or more atoms combine, they form a molecule.

If a molecule is composed of more than one element, it is a compound.

Cells are the smallest independent units of life. Some of the basic functions of cells are metabolism, irritability, growth and reproduction.

Tissues are composed of many similar cells that perform a specific function. Tissues are classified into four types, epithelial, connective, muscle and nervous. An organ is an integrated collection of two or more kinds of tissues that combine to perform a specific function. A system is a group of organs that work together to perform a major body function. All the body systems are specialized within themselves and coordinated with each other to produce an organism.

Body system

The integumentary system consists of the skin and all the structures derived from it. The main function of the skin is to protect the internal organs from the external environment.

The skeletal system consists of bones, certain cartilages and membranes and joints. It supports the body, protects the organs, enables the body to move, manufactures blood cells in the bone marrow and stores usable calcium and phosphorus.

The muscular system consists of the central nervous system and the peripheral nervous system. It also includes special sensory organs. The nervous system and the endocrine system are the body's main control and regulatory systems.

The endocrine system consists of a group of ductless glands that secrete hormones. Hormones regulate metabolic reactions within cells, growth and development, stress and injury responses, reproduction and many other critical functions.

The cardiovascular system consists of the heart, blood and blood vessels. An important function of the cardiovascular system is to transport oxygen and other necessary substances throughout the body and to transport wastes to the lungs and kidneys for removal.

The lymphatic system consists of lymph nodes, lymph and lymphatic vessels. It returns excess fluid and proteins to the blood and helps to protect the body from foreign substances, organisms and cancer cells.

The respiratory system accomplishes the process of breathing and provides a mechanism for the exchange of gases between blood and air.

The digestive system breaks down food physically and chemically into molecules small enough to be absorbed from the small intestine into the blood stream or lymphatic system. It also removes solid, undigested wastes.

The urinary system eliminates wastes produced by cells and regulates fluid balance in the body.

The production systems have organs that produce specialized reproductive cells that make it possible to maintain the human species.

The body cavities house and protect the internal organs. The two main body cavities are the dorsal and the ventral. The ventral body cavity is separated by the diaphragm into the superior thoracic and inferior abdominopelvic cavities. The dorsal cavity contains the cranial and spinal cavities.

The membranes line body cavities and cover or separate certain regions, structures and organs. The main types of membranes are mucous, serous and synovial.

Matter, elements and atoms

Matter is anything that occupies space and has mass. Mass refers to the amount of matter in an object. Matter is composed of elements, basic substances that cannot be broken down into simpler substances by ordinary chemical means. The atom is the smallest unit of an element that retains the chemical characteristics of that element.

Some of the elements critical to proper body function are oxygen, carbon, hydyogen, nitrogen, calcium and phosphorus.

The nucleus of an atom contains positively charged protons and uncharged neutrons. Orbiting the nucleus are negatively charged electrons.

Water is an inorganic compound. Organic compounds always contain carbon and hydrogen. Carbohydrates are made of carbon, hydrogen and oxygen with hydrogen and oxygen in a 2:1 ratio. They are an important source of energy.

The cell theory states that (a) all living organisms are composed of cells and products, (b) cell is the basic unit of structure and functions in all living organisms, (c) all cells come from the division of pre-existing cells and (d) an organism as a whole can be understood through the collective activities and interactions of its cellular units. All cells have four basic parts: the nucleus, nucleoplasma, cytoplasma and plasma membrane. Nucleus is the control centre of the cell. The nucleus contains the chromosomes that direct the production of and contain the genetic blueprint for new cells. The nucleus is surrounded by a nuclear envelope and contains nucleoplasma. The portion of the cell surrounding the nucleus is cytoplasm. The plasma membrane forms the outer boundary of the cell.

Cellular metabolism: The chemical processes that transform food into living tissue and energy are part of the body's metabolism, which includes all the chemical reactions in a living organism.

When cells divide more frequently than normal and do not die after the typical number of divisions, they form abnormal growth of tissue called a neoplasm. The cells of a benign neoplasm grow abnormally but do not differ significantly in structure from those in normal tissue and do not spread beyond their original site. The cells in a malignant neoplasm, cancer cells spread beyond the primary neoplasm and the establishment of secondary neoplasms in other parts of the body is called metastasis. The main categories of carcinogens (cancer causing agents) are chemical radiation and viruses. It is thought that most cancers are caused by repeated and prolonged exposures to the combination of several carcinogens. The main treatment for cancer are surgery, radiation therapy and chemotherapy. Combination therapy uses more than one type of therapy to treat cancer.

Endocrine glands do not have ducts. They release their secretions into the bloodstream. Exocrine glands release their secretions into ducts. Cartilage is a specialized connective tissue that provides support and facilitates movement at the joint. Nervous tissue is composed of several different types of cells, including neurons (impulse-conducting cells), non-conducting neuralgia and peripheral glial cells. Membranes are thin, pliable layers of epithelial or connective tissues that line body cavities, cover surfaces or separate or connect certain regions, structures or organs of the body.

Skin: Skin is the major part of the integumentary system, which includes hair, nail and glands of the skin. The epidermis of the skin is the outermost layer of epithelial tissue and dermis is the thicker layer of connective tissue beneath the epidermis. The hypodermis or subcutaneous layer lies beneath the dermis.

The dermis is composed of the thin papillary layer and the deeper, thicker reticular layer. Skin serves as a stretchable protective shield and is also involved in the regulation of body temperature; the excretion of waste materials and the synthesis of vitamin D3. It screens out harmful ultraviolet of the pigments melanin and carotene and the colour of underlying blood. Blood is supplied to the skin from blood vessels in reticular layer of the dermis. The wound healing process involves the formation of blood clots. Glands of the skin are sweat glands and the oil glands. Sweat glands are either eccrine glands (small sweat glands) that secrete sweat or apocrine glands which become active at puberty and produce thicker secretions. The major role of sweat glands is temperature regulation, while the main function of oil glands is lubrication.

Hair: Hair is composed of keratinized threads of cells that develop from the epidermis. Because of its embryonic origin, hair is considered to be an appendage of the skin. Hair consists of epithelial cells arranged in three layers, from the inside, out of a hair shaft. These are medulla, cortex and cuticle. The hair shaft protrudes from the skin, the root is embedded beneath the skin, and the entire structure is enclosed within a follicle. Human hair is constantly being shed and replaced. Hair follicles alternate between growing and resting phases.

Nails: Nails like hair are modifications of the epidermis. Composed of hard keratin nails are flat, keratinized plates on the dorsal surface of the distal segment of the fingers and toes.

During old age the skin usually becomes less elastic and more wrinkled, brittle and infection-prone. Uneven pigmentation may lead to blotched skin colour. Baldness in men and facial hair growth in women is common. All mature skin layers are present at birth. The first hairs begin to develop during 3rd fetal month. Terminal hairs appear at puberty in the genital area and armpit, and young men also develop chest and facial hair. Toe-nails and fingernails begin to develop at about 10th week of fetal development.

Bones: Bones are classified according to their shape as long, short, flat, irregular or sesamoid. Accessory bones are a minor category. Most long bones consist of a tubular shaft called diaphysis with an epiphysis at either end of the bone. The shapes of bones are related to their functions. The mechanical functions of bones include support, protection and movement. The epiphyseal plates and metaphyses are the only places long bones continue to grow in length after birth.

Bone (osseous) tissue is composed of cells embedded in a matrix of ground substance, inorganic salts, collagenous fibres. The inorganic salts give bone its hardness and the organic fibres and ground substance give it strength and flexibility. Most bones have an outer shell of compact bone tissue surrounding spongy bone tissue.

Bones contain 5 types of cells: Osteogenic cells which can be transformed into osteoblasts which synthesize and secrete new bone matrix as needed. Osteocytes help to maintain homeostasis. Osteoclasts, giant cells responsible for resonance of bone. Bone-lining cells have several diverse functions. Bone cells change their roles as the needs of the body change in growing and adult skeletons. Bones develop through ossification. Bones grow in diameter as osteogenic cells deposit new bone tissue beneath the periosteum and old bone tissue erodes. The growth of the diameter of bone continues through most of life. Bones help maintain homeostasis by strong calcium and other minerals to maintain proper levels of these minerals in the blood and other tissues. Red bone marrow produces red blood cells and white blood cells help fight disease. Several hormones have direct effect on bones and bones have effect on hormone secretion. Calcium and phosphorus make up about half of the content of bone. They must be supplied in a well balanced diet. Adequate levels of vitamins A, C & D are essential for the proper growth, mending and strength of bones. Aging bone become brittle from loss of calcium, decreased calcium utilization and decreased ability to produce matrix material. Skeletal problems affect women usually because of decrease in estrogen. The skeleton supports the body. It protects the inner organs and passage ways and acts as a system of levels that allows us to move.

The markings on the surface of a bone are related to the bone's function. Outgrowths on bones, openings to bones are the features of the bones. The skeleton (206 bones) is divided into 2 major portions: 80 axial skeletons (bones); 126 (bones) appendicular skeletons. They are joined together at the pectoral girdle and petric girdle to form the overall skeleton. The axial skeleton forms longitudinal axis of the body. It is made up of the skull, vertebral column, sternum and ribs. The appendicular skeleton is composed of the upper and lower extremities which include the pectoral and petric girdles. Each upper extremity consists of the pectoral girdle, upper arm bone, two form arm bones, wrist and hand bones. Each lower extremity consists of the petric girdle, upper leg bone, two lower leg bones, the ankle and foot bones. The skull is the skeleton of the head. It is divided as cranial skull and facial skull. The skull protects the brain, eyes, and provides points of attachment for muscles involved in eye movements, chewing, swallowing and other movements, and supports the mouth, pharynx and larynx. Except the ear orsicles and hyoid, the skull bones are joined together by seamlike joints that make the bones of an adult skull immovable. These are 8 cranial bones and 4 fontanels.

Frontal bones are 4 pairs of air cavities. There are 14 facial bones. Vertebral column or spine is the skeleton of the back. It is composed of 26 separate bones called vertebrae. The vertebral column protects the spinal cord and nerves, supports the weight of the body and keeps the body erect. Intervertebral disks act as shock absorbers and protect the vertebrae. The adult vertebral column has 4 curves which provide spring and resiliency. The processes of spinal vertebrae are attachment sites for muscles and ligaments. Cervical vertebrae are 7 between the skull and thorax. 12 thoracic vertebrae articulate with the ribs. 5 lumbar vertebrae are the largest and strongest vertebrae and provide attachments for lower back muscles. The adult sacrum which is composed by 5 fused vertebral bodies supports both the spinal column and the pelvis. The coccyx consists of 3 to 5 fused vertebrae.

The thorax is formed by the bodies and intervertebral disks of 12 thoracic vertebrae posteriorly, 12 pairs of ribs and 12 costal cartilages and the sternum anteriorly. The thoracic cage protects inner organs, provides a point of attachment for some bones and the muscles of the upper extremities, and provides a flexible breathing mechanism. There are 12 pairs of ribs, all of which articulate posteriorly with the vertebral column. The true ribs (1 to 7) attach to the vertebrae and sternum, 8-9-10 attach directly to the vertebral column and 11 & 12 are floating ribs as they are not even directly attached to the sternum or ribs above. The typical rib is composed of a head, neck and shaft.

The upper link of the appendicular skeleton includes the scapula and clavicle of the pectoral girdle, the humerus of arm, the radius and alma of the forearm, the carpel bone of the wrist, the metacarpels of the palm and the phalanges of the fingers. The main functions are: while the body moves, balancing; grasping of objects and manipulation of objects. Wrist has 8 carpels, palm has 5 metacarpels, thumb has two phalanges and each finger has 3 phalanges.

The lower limb consists of the bones of pelvic girdle, femur of thigh, tibia and fibula of the foreleg, tarsal of bones of the ankle, 5 metatarsals of the foot and 14 phalanges of toes and 1 patella. The functions are walking, balancing and standing. The pelvis is formed by sacrum, coccyx and hip bones. Female pelvis is lighter and wider than that of males as she has to carry and deliver a baby. The arches of the foot provide strength and resiliency. The transverse arch contacts the ground on one side only.

Bones give the body the structural framework and muscles give power; but joints (articulations) provide the mechanism that allows the body to move; immovable joints (synarthrosis), slightly movable (amphiarthrosis) and freely movable (diarthrosis). Structural classification of joints is fibrous, cartilaginous and synovial. The synovial joints are composed of the synovial cavity, articular cartilage, articular capsule and ligaments.

Types of synovial joints are 1. Hinge joints are uniaxial. 2. Pivot joints are uniaxial that have a rotational movement around a long axis through the centre of pivot. 3. Condyloid joints are like ball and socket with ligaments and muscles limiting movement to only two axes of rotation. 4. Gliding (plane) joints are small biaxial formed by essentially flat surfaces. 5. Saddle joints are multiaxial where both articulation bones have saddle shaped concave and convex areas. Ball and socket joints are most movable. Globe-like ball of one bone fits into the cup-like concavity (socket) of another.

Joint movements require stimulation by sensory and motor nerves which must have a ready blood supply. Sensory nerve fibres in joints relay information about joint activity to the spinal cord and brain, where it is processed and conveyed by nerve fibres to muscle controlling movement. Joints are nourished by blood vessels and drained of excessive tissue fluids by phatic vessels.

. Jaw (temporomandibular) joint is the only movable joint on head, (multiaxial) synovial joint, shoulder (glenohumeral) joint a multiaxial ball-socket joint. The head of the humerus articulates with shallow glenoid cavity of the scapula.

Hip (coxa) joint is multiaxial ball & socket synovial joint. Knee (tibiofemoral) joint is largest and complex and the weakest joint in the body. It is a synovial modified hinge joint. With age synovial fluid usually decreases, articular cartilage becomes thinner and ligaments become short and less flexible. Arthritis and other joint diseases become prevalent.

Muscles: The basic properties of muscle tissues are contractibility, excitability, extensibility and elasticity. And the functions are movement, posture and heat production. The three types of muscle tissues are skeletal, smooth and cardiac. Skeletal is striated muscle as it appears to be striped and voluntary muscle as it can be contracted voluntarily.

Skeletal muscle tissue is composed of individual cells, muscle fibres. Smooth muscle tissue is known as involuntary muscle. Cardiac muscle tissue is only in the heart which is involuntary. Cardiac muscle cells are closely attached end to end but remain separate. Cardiac muscle depends on nervous impulse to some extent, but it can contract rhythmically on its own. It can resist wear as it pumps blood continuously. With aging muscles become weaker, smaller and dehydrated. Reflexes slow and cramps may occur. Elderly people are less physically active with cardiac, vascular, digestive and respiratory problems.

A muscle is attached by a tendon to a bone or cartilage. Tendons add length and thickness to muscles, reduce muscle strain and add strength to muscle action. The origin and the insertion of some muscles can be reversed depending on which bone moves. The fibres of skeletal muscles are grouped into small bundles (fascicles) with the fibres within each bundle running parallel to each other. Most skeletal muscle movements are accomplished through a system of levers which include lever arm that pivots around a fixed point is fulcrum with bone acting as lever arm and joint as fulcrum.

Chapter 8

PANCAKARMA IN A NUTSHELL

Pancakarma, an ancient recognized therapeutic procedure, has great importance in Ayurveda. This therapy radiates the diseases and leaves no chance for relapse. This treatment has two functions: (i) it lightens the body and (ii) it nourishes the body. The lightening therapy is purificatory. It is pacifying and palliating the excess humours.

Pancakarmas are: Vamana (emesis), Virecana (purgation), Nasya or Shirovirecana (sternutation), Niruha basti (decoction enema) and Anuvasana basti (oily enema). Susruta considers both basti as one and adds Rakta Moksha (bloodletting) as the fifth.

If these therapies are administered properly, it will be helpful to cure by Ayurvedic treatment.

For easy elimination of humours, preliminary therapies are administered during each and every process. They are mainly (a) snehana (oleation) and (b) swedana (fomentation or sweating).

Oleation includes internal (drinking medicated oils or medicated ghee) and external (oil massage, oil bath, using oil on head etc.).

Internal oleation is generally done before emesis and purgation.

Sweating or fomentation includes touching with the heated solids, steam bath, massage with heated rice or leaf bundles.

Post-operation therapies are also mentioned after each process such as special diet, smoking with medicated fumes, gargling etc.

Oleation drugs have the following properties: heavy, cold, moving, unctuous, non-penetrating, minute, soft and liquid.

The main drugs are clarified butter, bone marrow, fat of animals and oil. Internal oleation is through mouth (drinking) and through anus (as enema). There are four types of external oleation: (i) Abhyanga, (ii) Seka, (iii) Sirobasti, (iv) Picu.

Oleation makes the boby unctuous and improves the flow of humours by liquefying them. It also softens the channels of humours and hence it promotes the elimination of humours. Oleation produces unctuousness, softness and regulates the flow of fluids inside the body.

Process and dosage of internal oleation: (a) only medicated oleation without food and drink, (b) medicated oils/clarified butter with rice, rice soup, meat soup, milk etc., in the form of enema, errhines, oil massage and retaining oil or ghee in the eyes. Dosage: (a) Minimum—the quantity which can be digested in six hours. (b) Medium—that can be digested in twelve hours and

(c) Maximum—the quantity which can be digested in twenty-four hours.

Internal oleation can be administered to: 1. after sudation, 2. after elimination, 3. who indulge more in liquors, 4. who indulge more in sex, 5. who indulge more in exercise, 6. who think too much, 7. the aged, 8. children, 9. debilitated, 10. emaciated, 11. who are dry, 12. anaemic, 13. reduced semen, 14. most of the diseases of wind (vata), 15. cataract and 16. difficulty in opening eyes soon after awakening.

Internal oleation is prohibited to: 1. very weak, 2. very strong, 3. who has excessive digestive fire, 4. very obese, 5. very emaciated, 6. stiffness in the thigh, 7. diarrhea, 8. presence of Ama, 9. throat diseases, 10. poisoning, 11. ascites (enlargement of abdomen), 12. nausea and vomiting, 13. excess mucus, 14. intoxication, 15. abnormal delivery and 16. after errhines and purgation.

Process of internal oleation:

Oleation should be taken before emesis and purgation. Proper time is after digestion of previous food and before the onset of appetite.

Patient's digestive fire should be checked to know the tolerance and reaction. There should not be any sign of ama. Before internal oleation, pass the urges and if necessary have bath.

First day small dose may be given. Close the eyes during drinking and burn incense for nice fragrance.

Following it, hot water should be consumed for its easy digestion and clearing the mouth from its coating. Covering the body the patient should lie down waiting for the digestion of oleation.

Signs during digestion: Headache, giddiness, nausea, fainting, weakness of the body, excessive thirst, burning sensation and anorexia (tastelessness).

Signs after digestion: After the above symptoms disappear: lightness of the body, free movement of wind (vata), onset of appetite, onset of thirst and clear belching.

Restrictions during internal oleation: 1. Food should be liquid, warm, not producing excess mucus in the body, not more fatty, nor a combination of various preparations. Food should be consumed in limited quantities on the previous day, during the period of oleation and a day after the oleation is stopped. 2. Warm water should be used for washing, bath, drinking etc. 3. Keep celibacy. 4. Sleep only at night. 5. Avoid (a) exercises, (b) exposure to cold breeze and sunlight, (c) anger and grief, (d) travelling, (e) long walk, (f) long speech or talk, (g) sitting for long time, (h) use normal pillow (not low, nor high) and (i) no contact with smoke and dust.

Generally the above restrictions are applicable to all treatments. These restrictions should be followed for the same number of days after the treatments.

Signs of proper internal oleation: (a) unctuousness of whole body, (b) oily stools, (c) oily skin, (d) softness of the body, (e) improved digestive fire, (f) free movement of wind (vata), (g) aversion towards oils, (h) general weakness of body and (i) more loose stool in consistency. Stop internal oleation when the above signs are found.

Patients having mild kostha (viscera abdomen) proper 3 days internal oleation is suggested; for medium kostha 5 days and for hard kostha 7 days.

Bad effect of improper internal oleation: less or excess dosage, improper time, improper food and improper activities of the patient produce bad effect. The main problems are: 1. Indigestion, 2. Excessive thirst,

3. Unconsciousness, 4. Distension of abdomen, 5. Fear, 6. Stiffness of body, 7. Anorexia, 8. Bodyache and 9. Formation of ama. Besides the following diseases, may have skin diseases, anaemia, oedema, ascites, diarrhea and piles.

For less oleation do the treatment again and for excess oleation give food and medicines which have opposite effect.

Benefits of internal oleation are: 1. Very keen digestive activity, 2. Clear alimentary tract, 3. Well developed tissue elements, 4. Improved physical strength, 5. Improved complexion, 6. Powerful sense organs, 7. Slow aging and 8. Increased life span.

SWEDANA (SUDATION)

Sudation removes the obstruction in the channels, removes stiffness, heaviness and cold of the body with sweating.

Oleation renders the body soft, disintegrates and liquefies the accumulated excreta. Sudation melts the toxins of the minute channels and thus brings them to viscera (Kostha).

Qualities of herbs for sudation: hot, sharp, moving, oily, subtle, liquid, steady, rough and heavy.

Classification of sudation: 1. Direct contact with heated materials, 2. Without direct contact of heat, such as exercise, without ventilation, covering with thick cloth, fear, sitting in the sunlight, drinking hot water in excess, application of hot drug-paste, fighting, anger and fasting.

Oily sudation for vata diseases and dry sudation for diseases of mucus.

Sudation can be locally and also for the whole body. According to potency there are mild, medium and strong sudation. Heated solid materials, paste of drugs, warm rice or leaf bundles and steam are generally used for sudation. Pouring warm liquids, hot hip bath and spinal bath etc. are also for sudation.

Sudation is indicated in the following diseases—cough, asthma, running nose, hiccup, hoarseness of voice, vata (wind) diseases, diseases of mucus, ama diseases, stiffness of body, heaviness of body, bodyache (whole or parts), constipation, tetanus, sprains, dysuria, tumours, urine obstruction, semen obstruction and stiffness of thighs.

Contraindications are: obese, weak, unconsciousness, injury to chest, emaciated, chronic, alcoholic, cataract, ascites, skin diseases just after taking milk, yoghurt, fat and honey, soon after elimination treatment, angry, fearful, jaundice, anaemia, diabetes, bile diseases, during menstruation and soon after delivery.

Process of sudation: Sudation is after internal or external oleation. It should be in a room devoid of cold breeze. The previous food be digested, but the patient should not feel excessive hunger. Eyes and heart should be protected from sudation.

Signs of proper sudation: Appearance of sweat, diminution of cold in the body, diminution of pain in the body and softness of body.

Never expose the body soon after sudation. Massage the body gently. Bathe in warm water after sudation. Obey the restrictions mentioned.

By excess sudation the patient may feel aggravation of bile and blood, thirst, loss of consciousness, giddiness, pain in joints, fever, black or red patches on skin and vomiting.

VOMITING

Vomiting eliminates humour of mucus through mouth. Along with mucus, a quantity of bile will be expelled from stomach. Vomiting is good to normal persons for keeping healthy during Vasanta.

To induce vomiting the drugs should have the following qualities: (a) hot potency and suddenly spreading; (b) subtle and sharp; (c) detachment, separates humours from their sites and takes to abdomen; (d) upward movement. It takes the humours upwards and expells from stomach through mouth.

Vomiting is administered in case of recent fever, diarrhea, bleeding piles, blood with stool and urine, pulmonary tuberculosis, leprosy and other skin diseases, diabetes, goitre, tumours, filariasis, insanity, cough, dyspnoea, herpes zoster, diseases of head.

Contraindications: Pregnant lady, more dry, excessive hunger, grief, aged, children, emaciated, obese, cardiac diseases, injury, debilitated, bouts of vomiting, spleen enlargement, cataract, worm infestation, giddiness, bodyache and diseases of vata.

Process of vomiting: The patient should be ready with internal oleation and sudation just a day before vomiting. Feed him the food containing black gram, sesame, fish, yoghurt etc. to produce more mucus by liquefying so that the humours would be expelled out.

In summer after oleation and sudation, a day before emesis, food for aggravating mucus is served. Next morning after passing the natural urges the patient sits on a chair facing east ready to drink a small quantity of rice soup adding clarified butter. According to the disease he drinks milk, sugarcane juice, meat soup or wine to the maximum capacity of the stomach.

Considering the bowel, digestive fire and the disease, the selected emetic drug sanctified with mantras is administered in the presence of experienced doctor. Wait 48 minutes with appearance of oppression in the chest, excessive salivation and nausea. The patient begins to vomit. If the bouts are not coming out easily he has to tickle his throat either with his fingers or with a soft tube without injuring the throat. Both the flank and forehead should be supported by another when bouts are coming up. His umbilical region and back be massaged in upward direction. Let him vomit till bile juice begins to come out or there is complete expulsion of mucus. If the bouts are insufficient, let him drink boiled water with long pepper, amalaki, mustard and salt.

Signs of proper vomiting: Mucus, bile and wind come out in successive order easily. He feels at ease and calm of mind and the bouts stop on their own accord.

If the vomitus is frothy, with blood, if he feels more weakness, burning sensation, dryness of throat, giddiness which are powerful diseases of wind origin, these are the signs of excess vomiting. Death due to discharge of blood also may happen.

Care after vomiting: Consolation after vomiting is a must. Let him inhale smoke and follow the regimen as in oleation.

First diet must be thin gruel. Thick gruel, rice with vegetable soup, rice with processed vegetable soup are the diet in successive order.

Humours are liquefied and their water element increases and reaches in the alimentary tract which reduces digestive fire. For improving digestive fire light diet is suggested.

Mild vomiting 4 bouts, 6 bouts medium and 8 bouts strong.

PURGATION

Purgation is the process of elimination of bile humour through anus. It is also a treatment for bile-mucus combination and mucus situated in the seat of bile. It is also good for vata.

Triphala, latex of hedged plant, castor oil etc. are the drugs for purgation. The qualities and actions of the drugs are—hot potency, penetrating, subtle, suddenly spread, detach humour from tissue elements and take humour downward and expell it through anus.

Fatty drugs: Castor oil, medicated ghee etc.

Non-fatty drugs: Haritaki, Triphala, grapes, latex of hedged plant. Benefit for—tumours of abdomen, piles, skin diseases, jaundice, chronic fever, ascites, poisoning, vomiting, disorders of spleen, abscesses, blindness, cataract and other eye diseases, pain in lower part of the body, genital disease, intestinal parasites, wounds/ulcers, gout, bleeding diseases of upward trend, blood diseases, obstruction of urine and faeces, diabetes, swelling and cough and dyspnoea.

Contraindications: Recent fever, less digestive power, bleeding downward, bouts, wounds, intestine ulcer, diarrhea, foreign matters in intestine, hard bowel movement, excess oleation and more emaciated.

Process: After oleation and sudation properly for three days, give food which does not aggravate mucus. The following day drugs for purgation may be given, soon after sunrise. Following give warm water to drink. Rest waiting for the bouts. After 1–2 normal bouts follow bouts with watering stools. Warm water should be drunk in between bouts. Sign of proper purgation is expulsion of mucus at the end and stopping purgation spontaneously.

Discomfort in chest and abdomen, anorexia, excessive salivation and spitting of mucus, itching and burning sensation and eruptions of skin, rhinitis and non-elimination of flatus and faeces are the signs of inadequate bouts.

Signs of excess bouts: After elimination of bile, mucus and wind in succeeding order, fluid resembling the water in which meat has been washed, expell fluid with fat, prolapse of rectum, excessive thirst, giddiness, bleeding through anus and if proper treatment is not given death may occur. After purgation diet is as for vomiting.

STERNUTATION

Nasal medication or sternutation is otherwise called Sirovirecana. Generally it benefits all the three humours and is specially effective for vata (wind) and mucus. The excess humours accumulated in the head, throat, nose and sinus are removed by this treatment. As the life force enters through nostrils and controls the functions of cerebrum, sensory and motor functions of the body, the drugs administered through them reach all over the head including throat and upper part of the chest and collect the excess humours and expell through mouth.

Sternutation is classified as elimination, nourishing and palliating or curing. Eliminating treatment is indicated in headache, heaviness of head, throat diseases, swelling, enlargement of salivary glands, worms, tumours, skin diseases, epilepsy and rhinitis. Medicated oil, ghee, decoctions or pastes which expell mucus are used for treatment.

Nourishing is indicated in vata (wind) originated headache, hoarseness of voice,dryness in mouth and nose, difficulty in speaking or opening the eyes or movements of arms. Medicated oil having nourishing property, juice of meat/meat soup are used for the treatment. Hair and eye diseases, discoloured patches of skin etc. are treated as palliating/curing by using the medicated oil, decoctions, milk or water.

Minimum dose is 6 bindu (1 bindu is the quantity of liquid that blows down after immersing 2 digits of the index finger and taking it out). Medium is 8, and maximum is 10. To the wounded, emaciated, children and aged the smaller dose is 2 bindus.

Sternutation with paste is applied by pressing or squeezing the medicated paste. Medicated powders are administered by blowing inside the nostrils with the help of air from the mouth the powder in a tube about 6 inches (15 cm) long having both ends open. Inhalation of fumes/ smoke with medicated fumes is also given.

Contraindications: Cough, dyspnoea, vomiting, hiccup, acute rhinitis, just consumed water/liquor/poison/ oil, after bath, after bloodletting therapy, ladies recently delivered, after vomiting and purgation and basti (enema) therapies and when the sky is more cloudy.

Process: After passing the natural urges apply oil to the upper portion of the shoulders and forehead close to the eyes while sudation to the head. Let the patient lie down face up in a room devoid of breeze, stretching the arms and legs (legs slightly raised) and head lowered so that the nostrils will be upward. Slightly warm the medicine and using the dropper instill into each nostril alternately keeping the other closed. After instillation massage his soles, palms, neck, shoulders, cheeks, nose and forehead. Let him turn to his sides and spit out till entire medicine comes out. If he faints, sprinkle cold water over him (except head). Let him rest 5 minutes and gargle the mouth with lukewarm water.

By proper treatment the patient gets easy expiration, sleep, easy awakening and clarity of sense organs.

Sternutation is prohibited to children under 7 years and the aged over 80 years.

By sternutation shoulders, chest, neck, face and skin become bright; sense organs become strong. Habitual sternutation protects from early greying.

BASTI (ENEMA)

There are three kinds of enema: (1) oil enema, (2) decoction enema and (3) enema through urethra/vagina.

Benefits for diseases: Tumour, tympanitis, gout, arthritis, spleen diseases, diarrhea without ama, abdominal colics, chronic fever, flowing nose, obstruction of semen, flatus and faeces, enlargement of scrotum and diseases of wind (vata) origin.

Contraindications: Excess oleation therapy, chest injury, highly emaciated, diarrhea with ama, vomiting, dyspnoea, cough, piles, weak digestion, swelling of rectum soon after food, intestinal obstruction, perforation and pregnancy till 8th month.

Benefits of oil enema: Oil enema is powerful in extreme dryness and uncontrolled digestive fire.

Contraindications for oil enema: Anaemia, jaundice, diabetes, rhinitis, lack of food, spleen diseases, diarrhea, enlargement of abdomen, profound obesity, intestinal parasites, gout, having poison.

Basti instruments: Enema nozzle, enema bag. Nozzle with metal, upper end narrow, lower end wider having holes at both ends, straight and smooth. The bladder of goat, sheep, buffalo devoid of holes and tears be filled with drugs and tied tightly with lower part of nozzle.

Process of oil enema: 1. Oil massage. 2. Fomentation. 3. Bath. 4. Eat ¼ of usual food with proper liquid drink. 5. After elimination of the natural urges let him lie on his left side folding his right thigh and stretching the other. 6. Lubricate enema nozzle and rectum with ghee or oil and push into rectum. 7. Gently press the bag and push the medicine into colon. 8. Let him lie on his back and massage his abdomen, thigh and buttocks. 9. Let his legs be little up so that the medicine should not come out soon.

Maximum time for oil to come out is 9 hours. If oil does not come out due to excessive dryness of Kostha, it can be neglected. Oil enema can be administered daily to: 1. Profound increase of wind, 2. One who does exercise, 3. Who has keen digestive power and 4. Who is very dry.

Process of decoction enema: 180 gm honey, 15 gm rock-salt, oil/ghee, 180 gm pippalyadi, 150 gm satapushpa pounded, and decoction of ricinus.

Mix and churn honey and oil/ghee well, add pounded satapushpa and mix again and add decoction and mix the drug.

The drug should not be too thick or too thin. Fill the bag when the mix is lukewarm and tie tightly to the nozzle. Let the patient eliminate the faeces and lie on the back, face up.

Maximum time for decoction enema is 48 minutes. If it does not come out another purgative enema with alkaline (cow's urine) should be given. It will irritate sphincter and medicine will come out. If the medicine comes out soon, another basti with the same medicine can be given. After enema bathe with warm water. The diet should be rice with soup (meat soup also). Decoction for vata diseases should be pacifying, like sweet, sour and salty in taste and hot mixing with oil/ghee and rock-salt.

For bile the drugs should be sweet, cold mixed with ghee, milk, sugarcane juice and honey.

For mucus Aragwathadi is good. The drugs should be dry, hot and pungent mixing with honey, cow's urine etc.

Karma Basti: 30 enemas (in the beginning 1 oil enema, 5 oil enemas at the end; 12 decoction and 12 oil enemas alternately in the middle).

Kala Basti: 15 enemas (1 oil enema in the beginning, 3 oil enemas at the end, 6 decoction enemas and 5 oil enemas alternately in the middle).

Yoga Basti: 8 enemas (1 oil enema in the beginning and 1 oily at the end, 3 decoction with 3 oily alternately in the middle).

Matra Basti is for the aged and children.

Uttara Basti is for urinary and vaginal diseases. Dosage: 24 gm for male, 48 gm for female and 24 gm for children.

Chapter 9

SOME DISEASES AND THEIR TREATMENT

NASAL DISEASES

Diagnosis of causes of disease: 1. Exposure to mist, fog, wind and dust. 2. Excessive talk, very loud and/or for long time. 3. Using very high or very low pillow. 4. Drinking of water in violation of the norms (more quantity, when hungry, more cold, kept for several days in a vessel, contaminated, collected from unsuitable/unaccustomed area, without considering the season). 5. Excessive/untimely water sports. 6. Suppression of forceful natural urges connected to the area above the neck (such as suppression of vomiting, forceful/excessive vomiting, suppression of tears, forceful production/excessive shedding of tears, suppression of sneezing, forceful production/excessive sneezing).

All these aggravate vata (wind) which contaminates the other humours and lead them to accumulate in the area of nose. Thus catarrh or cold is produced.

Catarrh is divided according to the predominance and stage of progress as follows:

Vata (wind) Catarrh: Dryness of mouth/face, profuse sneezing, blockage of the nose and pricking pain, pain in the teeth, feeling of insect crawling in the area of eyebrows, discharge of clear and thin secretion from the nose are the main symptoms. Ripening will be slow.

Bile Catarrh: Feeling of thirst, fever, eruption inside the nose, dizziness, ulceration of mucous membrane at the tip of the nose, warm-yellowish-reddish-non-sticky discharge which gets dry soon.

Mucous Catarrh: Associated with cough, anorexia, dyspnoea, vomiting, heaviness of head, sweet taste in mouth, itching in the affected area. Nasal discharge will be white and viscous.

Catarrh due to aggravation of all the 3 humours: Mixed symptoms.

Blood Catarrh: Vitiated humours accumulated in the nasal area constantly communicate with the blood of that area and contaminate it. So blood catarrh is produced. Numbness and discomfort in the chest, copper coloured eyes, foul smelling breath, itching of nose, ears and eyes, and the symptoms of bile catarrh.

Improper management or negligence on all the above types leads to severe catarrh. The contamination of humours and tissue elements reflects on all parts of the body and impairs all physiological functions. Loss of appetite, indigestion, fever, dyspnoea, cough, chest pain, lateral sides pain, bad smell of mouth, foul smelling breath, feeling of dryness and blockage in the nose, pus-like discharge, black and red coloured nodular particles discharge from the nose and fainting. Finally worms will be developed.

When catarrh becomes ripened, disappear sneezing and profuse discharge. Feels lightness. Smell and taste are re-established.

Treatment: 1. The patient should keep away from all causes of disease. 2. Oleation, fomentation, vomiting, smoking fumes may be done according to the condition. 3. Neck and above the neck may be covered with wool cloth to keep warm. 4. Food and drink must be light, oily with sour and salty taste. 5. Liquid diet is also good.

Oral medicine: Vyoshadhi pills—peenasa, shurasa, kasa and aruci.

For smoking: Anethu sowa, cinnamomum zeylanicum, sida retusa or sida cordifolia, oraxylum indicum, ricinus communis, aegle marmalos and cassia fistula. These drugs are used for smoking along with muscle fat, ghee or beeswax according to the condition. Powdered poprice with ghee can also be used for smoking.

Bath, anger, excess sleep, day-sleep, cold water, cold food etc. should be avoided.

MENTAL DISEASES

Insanity is classified: 1. wind (Vata), 2. bile, 3. mucus, 4. aggravation of all the three humours, 5. due to grief and other physical disturbances, 6. poisons. Symptoms in all are alike. Purgatives and emollient treatment are given for wind, like mucus or all the three aggravated diseases.

Brahmi (Cleodendron indica) is the main drug used for treatment. It is a tonic stimulant and alternative. Ghee prepared with this is also good.

Epilepsy which is loss of consciousness is treated separately. Convulsive fits as hysteria etc. are also considered as mental diseases. Grief, fear, obsessive thinking etc. are the main reasons for this kind of diseases. The severe form of the fits is absent and is replaced by a momentary loss of consciousness, tremors and restlessness. Aura is also present. It is petite.

Pancagavya Ghrita or Mahapancagavya Ghrita, in which many of nervine tonic and sedative drugs are mentioned, is mainly used in both epilepsy and insanity. Pancagavya contains urea and its salts, unaltered biliary pigments, lactic acids and lactates etc. Urea has an antiperiodic and antispasmodic action.

FRACTURES AND DISLOCATIONS

Restriction of movement, pain and tenderness are the symptoms of dislocation.

Swelling and tenderness at the site of fracture, crepitus, abnormal mobility and discomfort in all postures are the symptoms of fracture.

Dislocations are classified into six according to the relative positions and fractures are classified into 12 varieties as comminuted, impacted, compound etc. There is chance of union if fracture and dislocation are properly attended to.

Cartilages only bend. Long bones break in twain, flat bones crack and small bones break into pieces.

Rocking movement, pressure, bringing together and bandage are the treatment. The deformity also should be corrected. If there is more swelling at the site of fracture or dislocation apply cloth dipped in medicated ghee. Wash with cold decoctions and apply splint when swelling is reduced.

Fracture of nasal bones is treated with two tubes open at both ends, inserting into the nostrils instead of splint.

In case of malunion better to break it again and treat it as fresh fracture. In compound fracture if the bone protrudes without the periosteum, that part may be cut off and treat as compound fracture. Compound fractures of cranium with escape of brain matter as well as similar punctured wounds, after cleaning, put in a cigarette drain made of hairs, the same as used for suturing and as the ulcer heals, it is recommended to remove the drain by a few hairs a day till complete healing. In other places such drain smeared with oily matter is recommended.

FISTULA IN ANO

There is some relation between fistula and ischiorectal abscess. In all cases operation is advised. The expert physicians do the treatment properly.

SURGERY IN AYURVEDA

All wounds and ulcers are classified as fresh and old. A wound for the first seven days, showing clearly healing, is called fresh wound. After that period it is known as ulcer, old ulcer, chronic ulcer etc. Ulcer means a dissolution of continuity of tissue. In any case the treatment constitutes an application of honey and ghee. Due to the large content of sugar honey acts as a lymphagogue exactly as hypertonic saline would do. The nutrient properties of honey help to promote granulation tissue. Due to the astringent content it has some astringent property as well. Ghee besides its emollient property tends to occlude the surface from contamination. Honey is mildly antiseptic also, due to its alcoholic content (autofomentation). So the first dressing is at once non-irritating (non-tissue destroying) with properties conducive to sterilisation of wound (by purely physiological means) and promotion of granulation.

Combat surgical conditions are: plasters, irrigation of wounds, ointments, fomenting, massage, warm poultices, measures to promote suppuration, blood letting and depletion of blood to counteract the venous stasis, excision, incision, scraping or removal of unhealthy tissue, extraction of foreign bodies causing irritation, puncturing and exploring, suturing, arresting of haemorrhage, dramage, application of mercurial remedies (antiseptic active methods), dusting of powders, fumigation (antiseptic measure), promoting granulation, destroying proud flesh, softening in duration, hardening the parts (as in impending bedsores), application of caustics for destruction of tissues, actual cautery, promoting pigmentation or colouring of the surface, removal of excessive pigmentation, grafting of living flaps, growing of hair, permanent epilation, enemate, bladder and vaginal douching, various bandagings, washing out of sinuses such as frontal, gargles, fumigation, various non-cutting surgical appliances and instruments (beds, splints, catheters, forceps etc.), sharp instruments, protection from psychosomatic measures. It is clear that they had all measures except radiological and similar aids.

Boiling the instruments before operations is also in Ayurveda. Fumigation with many materials has antiseptic virtues. Mercury and arsenical compounds are also used as antiseptics. Sugar solution is as good as hypertonic saline. Among hypertonic saline, saturated Mag Sulph solution and sugar solution are the best.

In Ayurveda there is no mention about anaesthesia except to doping alcohol. The ancient physicians had the knowledge about some marma points where they used to press and the patient became unconscious. When the treatment is over they would press another point by which the patient would regain his consciousness. There were some herbal powders which were used for smelling, by which the patient would be unconscious. There were four pillars of surgery in Ayurveda: anatomy, anaesthesia, asepsis and some form of antiseptic, and methods of arresting haemorrhage.

There was plastic surgery of various forms. Rhinoplastic and plastic operations on the earlobes were quite satisfactory.

In place of transfusion of blood in serious cases blood was administered orally.

Ancient physicians knew the dangers of leaving a foreign body in the wound and hence the removal of it was strongly advocated. The wealth of surgical armamentarium has been ably treated.

OBSTETRICS AND GYNAECOLOGY IN INDIAN MEDICINE

Ayurvedic physicians of yore had a clear concept of obstetrics and gynaecology. Descriptions of various diseases of women and their treatments are found in the treatises on internal medicine. Embryology, ante-natal care and care of pregnant women during and after labour are dealt with along the anatomy and physiology of the genital tract. The gynaecological conditions are mentioned along with the internal medicine.

Ante-natal care is given sufficient emphasis in specialised treatises. During the development of the foetus at every stage the ante-natal care is also mentioned. The ante-natal care can be divided into: 1. Hygiene of the pregnant women, 2. Dietetics. The pregnant woman has to lead a peaceful and religious life. She should never indulge in exhaustive exercise and should observe celibacy. The dress should be very light and loose around the waist. Use of heavy blankets is also prohibited. Day-time sleep, awaking till late at night, sitting on hard surface and unwholesome habits are contraindicated. Fasting and long walk are also not good. Should have regular bowels.

Diet should be appetising and nourishing, and rich in body building. But she should not have indgestion or fermentation.

To maintain mental hygiene she should be happy and all her desires should be fulfilled. She should not have any mental shock.

Mostly liquid, non-spicy, relishing and tasty food is suggested for the first 3 months. During this period desire for food will be less and spicy food may cause more vomiting.

For the 4th month a diet rich in milk, butter and less in carbohydrates is suggested for preventing toxaemias of pregnancy.

During 5th, 6th and 7th months follow the same diet having minimum requirements of sodium chloride, acids and carbohydrates. Dietetics which act by increasing kidney function are also prescribed.

During 8th and 9th months diet containing high proteins and minerals is good. Avoid constipation, if necessary decoction enema can be applied. During 9th month for lubricating the passage tampons can be used.

Obstetrics: In Ayurveda the expulsion of fertilised ovum up to the 4th month is called 'Sravam' (abortion), till the end of 7th month miscarriage (Patan) and later 'Prasavam' (delivery).

Difficult labour: (1) If the foetus is dead, the patient is to be placed on the back with buttocks a little raised. With lubricated hand passing into the uterus the foetus is to be taken out. (2) If the child is alive: (a) Feet presentation—should be delivered as such by pulling out the feet—podalic delivery. (b) If single foot is presented, the other foot also be pulled out and then should be delivered as before. (3) In breech presentation, the buttocks are to be pushed up and converted into podalic presentation and delivered as before. (4) Transverse presentation: It should be treated by combined version, pushing up to breech and bringing down the vertex and delivered. (5) If head presents as sides, or face, or brow the shoulder should be pushed up and converted as vertex and delivered. (6) If hand prolapses, the hand and shoulder should be pushed up and converted as vertex and delivered. (7) Hands, legs and head may together present impacted. This cannot be delivered alive. (8) Craniotomy: The skull of the child is to be opened by a painted sharped piercing instrument. The skull bone should be wrenched out. With hook on chest or axilla, the foetus should be pulled out. If the head is not broken up the orbit or jaw could be used to hook the foetus down. Taking both descriptions into consideration it will be noted that hooking on chest or axilla was contemplated in the event of all head bones being removed. This is virtually decapitation. If the head is otherwise intact, pulling is to be done on orbit or jaw. Impacted shoulders and pelvic presentations, the limbs are to be amputated. If the abdomen is enlarged evisceration is recommended.

Dead foetus should on no account be permitted to remain in the womb. It should be removed immediately. The disorders of pregnancy are nausea and vomiting, oedema, fever, diarrhea, retention and suppression of urine. Convulsion is one of the disorders of pregnancy. The treatment is based upon (1) drugs used for symptomatic relief and (2) drugs to cure diseases, the importance of diet and preventive measures are stressed.

Treatment after delivery: Soon after delivery the lady is to be washed and cleaned. Milk prepared with sedatives is given for the first ten days. Her diet should be nourishing and light. From 11th day vegetable/meat soup and diet suitable to the constitution are suggested. Take care till 4th month. If the delivery is not natural (manual and instrumental manipulations), after cleaning the patient the vaginal canal is to be anointed with medicated oil. A decoction of Allizzia lebbeck and Terminala (both astringents) is recommended. Bala Taila should be used after 20 days. It is good in all nervous ailments and is general restorer of health. It acts as good ecbolic gynaecologically.

The causes of diseases of women's sexual orgán are: Excessive indulgence, menstrual derangements, use of self-abuse and dangers from the ovum.

Preparations of Asoka (Saracca indica) in the form of medicated ghee and decoction are suggested in all classics. Another common medicine is Pushyanaga powder which is generally given during excessive flow as it contains many drugs which are haemostatic and slypic. To increase health and vitality Satavari Ghee and Satavari Rasayanam are prescribed. Anaemia is treated with suitable iron preparations as Pradarantaka Rasam and Pradaradi Leham. Douching, fumigation and local warmth are also advised.

SPECIAL TREATMENTS OF KERALA

Some Ayurvedic treatments, in a traditional way, are known as Keraliya treatments. These treatments appear to have been built upon the classical Ayurvedic approach of "Purvakarma" component. (treatment done before conducting "Pancakarma", and some are post-operative, palliative treatments. Major special therapies are as follows.

Dhara (Flow): This is a process to trickle slowly the medicated oil, milk, ghee, butter decoction through Dhara Varti (Probe) on the forehead of the patient lying down below the Dhara pot hanged on an appropriate height on the Dhara table. The medicated liquid is selected according to the disease, constitution and other factors of the patient. It is very effective for diseases of eye, ear, nose and throat and also for palsy neuropathies, insomnia, loss of memory etc.

I just explain how buttermilk Dhara (Takra Dhara) is done. Take 90 gms of Musta, peel and pound it and make a bundle in a clean cotton cloth. Put the bundle in one litre of milk adding 4 litres of water. Boil it and reduce to one litre. Add 2 tablespoon yoghurt when the milk is lukewarm. Keep it 8 to 10 hours till the milk is turned into yoghurt. Remove butter by churning it.

Remove seeds from 1 kg of dried Amalaki and adding 4½ litre water in it boil and reduce to one litre. Strain it and make it cool. While churning if necessary a small quantity of this water can be added to remove the butter. When the buttermilk is ready mix this water in it.

Let the patient lie down on his back on the Dhara table. The Dhara pot having a hole in the bottom in which a cotton wick of thickness equal to small finger is hanged through the hole to make the liquid flow through the wick. It should be hanged at the required height above the head of the patient. The wick should be 3 inches (8 cm) above the forehead of the patient.

Tie a cloth above the eyebrows of the patient to prevent the flow towards the eyes. Fill the dhara pot with buttermilk and let the flow of it fall on the forehead of the patient. Move gently the dhara pot so that the flow may fall from one end of the forehead to another. Continue this 45 minutes without break of the stream. Collect the liquid flowing through the head for refilling the pot till the treatment is over. Fresh buttermilk is suggested for each day.

After the treatment the patient can bathe in warm water. Apply Rasnadi powder on head, and rub well.

Whole Body Fomentation/Pizhichil: Medicated oils or decoctions are poured all over the body of the patient from dhara pot, or cloth dipped in the liquid and simultaneously massage is done by which tissues are strengthened. It also promotes biological fire. The lustre and beauty of the body is enriched, ojas is stabilised, sense organs become clear and longevity is achieved. It also helps regeneration and rejuvenation of the body. By this therapy the patient gets the effect of oleation and also sudation together which is the best treatment for vata diseases.

The treatment room must be devoid of cold breeze with a table of which the surface should be convex with a hole at the lower end for collecting the medicated liquid applied on the patient.

The patient after passing the natural urges with empty stomach wearing a brief should sit on the table stretching the legs. Apply special oil on the head and paste of Amalaki over it. Four attendants/masseurs, 2 on both sides of the table, 1 above the hip and the other below the hip on each side—are for applying oil on the patient, and one attendant is for warming the oil. The paste of Amalaki is made with milk or buttermilk. According to the patient and the disease 1-1½ litre medicated oil daily is used for this treatment. Warm the oil keeping the temperature constant. Apply the warm oil on the whole body and massage for thirty minutes. The cotton cloth pieces (30 cm x 30 cm each x 4) are dipped in the warm oil and squeezed from a height of 20-25 cm with the right hand, then gently massage with the left hand. All the four masseurs massage the patient simultaneously. The flow of warm oil falls on the patient's body. The collected oil in the vessel kept below the table is warmed again and used. This procedure continues for about 90 minutes. Then the oil is wiped off. There are 7 postures for Pizhichil: (1) sitting with stretched legs; (2) lying on back; (3) lying on left side; (4) lying on stomach (back up); (5) lying on right side; (6) lying on back (as no. 2); (7) sitting (as no. 1). When the body is in the normal temperature the patient can bathe. After bath apply Rasnadi powder on the head and give Gandharva hastadi decoction internal for Vata.

The period of treatment is for 7 days, 14 days or 21 days according to the disease. During the treatment patient should follow the regimen as in internal oleation.

All vata diseases as hemiplegia, monoplegia, muscular contractures, wasting of muscles, arthritis, weak, emaciated and aged can be cured by this treatment.

Navarakkizhi or Rice Bundle Massage: Rice bundle massage is included in fomentation, though it is not sudation therapy but it is the best among nourishing therapies. Hence it is advised in all emaciating diseases and all chronic vata diseases. Prior to rice bundle treatment, adequate external oleation is necessary.

The decoction is prepared using 60 gms of Sida cordifolia (or any other drug according to the disease); adding 12 litre water, reduce it by boiling up to 3 litres. Add 1.5 litres of decoction in 1.5 litres of milk for cooking 360 gms of coarse rice. Cook the rice well so that while pressing it should be a paste. No liquid portion should be in the vessel after cooking. Divide the cooked rice into 4 equal parts and make bundles using the cotton cloth 30 cm x 30 cm for each. Holding the 4 corners together tie tightly with a strong string.

The patient should be with empty stomach. Let him sit on the treatment table. Put special oil on the head. Then massage the whole body, apply the prescribed oil properly for half an hour. Boil the rest of 1.5 litre decoction with 1.5 litre milk in a wide mouthed vessel. Keep the bundles inside the vessel so that the handle of the bundle should not dip in milk. Two masseurs taking one bundle each massage the patient's body with the bundle with tolerable heat. While massaging squeeze the rice out through the bundle. Out of three masseurs, one will be heating the bundles. When the bundles get cooled, they are changed with hot ones. Massage is only downward without more pressure but it should be done quickly when it is hot and when it is getting cooler massage slowly. This massage is done in 7 postures as in pizhichil. The duration of massage is 45 minutes to one hour. In the end whole content in the bundle is squeezed out and applied on the body. Finally the paste is scraped out of the body. Rub the body with a dry cloth. Massage with oil for 10 minutes and rest for another 10 minutes and bathe using warm medicated water.

In some diseases the cooked rice is applied directly without bundle and rub and massage the whole body, or any part. Such treatment is known as Njavara Tepu or Njavara Tirummal. The pinda sweda (bundle fomentation) is helpful to a great extent to the patients suffering from different neuromuscular disorders.

Sirolepa (Covering the Head with Paste): Mental and brain disorders are treated by applying medicated paste over the head of the patient. Thirunnavaya Moosad treated a crazy man who was in the mental hospital for 3 months, covering his head with the fresh cowdung. Keeping it for about an hour his head was washed with rice bran water. This treatment continued for three weeks with Brahmi Ghritam and a decoction for internal use. By this treatment he was 75% normal. Then the physician changed the oral medicine and with another two weeks' treatment the patient was completely normal.

Sirovasti (Retaining Oil on Head): Sirovasti is indicated in numbness of scalp, facial palsy, insomnia, dryness of nose, throat and mouth, migraine, headache, trinitus and other diseases of head.

After passing the natural urges, on empty stomach the patient is oleated all over the body following a mild fomentation. In the evening he sits on a stool of the height of the knee, a strap of leather (either of cow or buffalo) of 25 cm width and length equal to the circumference of the head should be wrapped around the head just above the ears, over a cotton cloth ribbon of 3 cm width fixed on the forehead with black soya paste. The joints and intervening spaces also should be packed with the paste of black soya. Medicated oil prescribed for the disease is poured over the head, in lukewarm condition to a height of 2.5 cm over the scalp. The duration of treatment (1) till secretion appears in the mouth and nose, (2) 53 minutes for Vata diseases, (3) 42 minutes for bile diseases, (4) 32 minutes for mucous diseases and (5) 5 minutes 30 seconds for healthy persons. It is necessary to retain the same temperature of the oil on the head. Hence when the oil gets cold remove little by little and refill with warm oil little by little. The removed oil can be warmed again for the day's use.

When the treatment is over remove the whole oil, the cap and the ribbon etc. and massage over shoulders, back, neck and forehead. Let him bathe in warm water. This treatment can be done for 3, 5 or 7 days.

Leaf Bundle Massage (Patra Potala Sweda): Cut the leaves of arka (calotropis), sigra (drumstick), chincha (tamarind), dhatoora (white thorn-apple) and nirgundi. Scrape half a coconut, cut the lemon into pieces. Putting neem (margo) oil in a wide mouthed vessel boil, put the leaf cuttings, lemon pieces and coconut scrapes and fry till the coconut scrapes get brownish red colour. Put the fried leaves in the middle of a cotton cloth (30 cm x 30 cm) and tie it well like a bundle. The size of the bundle will be the size of a medium coconut. Make 4 such bundles for treatment as rice-bundle-massage.

The massaging procedure is as rice-bundle-massage. The bundles are heated in the prescribed medicated oil according to the disease keeping it hot in the frying pan. The treatment is for 45 minutes.

This treatment is given to the patients of arthritis, numbness, tremor generalized, bodyache due to vata, hemiplegia and other vata diseases. Avoid this for bile and blood aggravated patients.

Instead of leaf bundle or rice bundle, various medicinal cereals coarse powder is used for applying on the body in the form of bundles. It is suggested for parasthasia, improper blood and lymphatic circulation and other vata diseases.

INDEX

A

Ama 35
  symptoms of association of malas and humours with 35-36
Ayurveda
  aims and objects of 11
  definition of 11
  eight branches of 12-14
  surgery in 139-141

B

Bath, effect of 63
Bile (Pitta), qualities of 28, 29
Bile humour
  signs of diminution of 38
  treatment of 40
Blood
  source of 73
Blood diminution
  treatment of 40
Bone marrow
  signs of diminution of 39
Bone tissue
  signs of diminution of 39
Breast milk
  signs of diminution of 40
Buffalo's milk, qualities of 23
Butter, qualities of 23
Buttermilk, qualities of 23

C

Camel milk, qualities of 23
Coconut water, qualities of 22
Cohabitation for offspring
  days suitable for 76-78
  postures to be adopted 77
Cold water, qualities of 22
Conception, process of 75-76
Constitution (prakriti), nature of 43-46
Cow's milk, qualities of 22
Curd, qualities of 23

D

Day and night
  examination of 55
  regimen of 62
Death
  prediction of 89-90, 105-108
  process of 85

Digestive fire 70-71
Disease diagnosis
- Chinese pulse examination 98-99
- eye test 103-104
- nail examination 105
- pulse examination 95-97
- stool test 102-103
- teeth examination 104-105
- Tibetan pulse examination 97-98
- tongue test 104
- urine test (Ayurveda) 99-102

Diseases
- categories of 16, 17-18
- characteristic features on which curability depends 15-16
- classification of by Susruta 17
- curable 17
- incurable 17
- transmigratable 16

Diseases caused by aggravation of bile 32-33
- symptoms of aggravation of bile 32
- treatment of 33-34

Diseases caused by aggravated mucus 34
- symptoms of aggravated mucus 34
- treatment of 34-35

Diseases caused by aggravation of wind 31
- symptoms of aggravation of wind 31-32
- treatment of 32

Dreams 91-94
Drugs
- astringent 49
- classification of, on the basis of therapeutic effect 48
- digestive 49-50
- earthy 48
- emetic 49
- inside the earth 48
- nourishing 49
- on the earth 48
- purgative 49
- role of 47
- sky 49
- types of 50-52
- watery 48
- windy 49

E

Epidemics (contagious)
- management of 61-62

Examination
- three types of 17

Excreta (Malas) 38, 72
- signs of diminution of 39
- treatment of 40

F

Fat
- signs of diminution of 39

Fermented rice water, qualities of 24
Fistula in ano
- treatment of 139

Flowers, effect of 63-64

Foetus
process of growth of 79-80
Food
digestive process of 71-72
favourable and avoidable 25-26
Fortnight, examination of 55
Fractures and dislocations
classification of 138
symptoms of 138
treatment of 139
Freshly conceived lady
characteristic features of 78-79

G

Goat's milk, qualities of 23
Gynaecology 141-143

H

Healthy person
attributes of 66-67, 86
Honey, qualities of 23
Hot water, qualities of 22
Human body
no. of marmas in 85
the states of 91
Human body—anatomy and physiology
atom to organism 109-110
body system 110-111
bones 115-119
cellular metabolism 112-113
hair 114
muscles 119-120
nails 114-115
skin 113-114

J

Joints, kinds of 84-85

K

Kerala, special treatments of 145-149
Dhara (flow) 145-146
leaf bundle massage 150
Navarakkizhi 147-149
Pizhichil 146-147
Sirolepa 149
Sirovasti 149-150

L

Land inhabited by patients
types of 42-43
Living creatures
sources of origin of 47

M

Matters (Dravyas)
movable 48
properties of 67-68
types of 47
Menstrual blood
properties of 73
signs of diminution of 40
source of 73
treatment of 41
Menstruation period
dos and don'ts for women during 76
Mental diseases
classification of 137-138
treatment of 138

Messengers' role to know the result of treatment 87-89
Mother's milk, qualities of 23
Mucus (Kapha)
- pains caused by vitiation of 38
- qualities of 28, 29
- signs of diminution of 39
- treatment of 40

Muscle tissue
- signs of diminution of 39

N

Nasal diseases 135-137
- treatment of 137

Nirma bile 36
Nirma wind
- symptoms of 35, 36

Nurse, qualities of 15

O

Obstetrics 143-145
Oils, qualities of 24
Ornaments, effects of 64

P

Pancakarma
- enema (Basti) 132-134
  - benefits of 132
  - contraindications 132-133
  - instruments 133
  - process of 133-134
  - kala 134
  - karma 134
  - matra 134
  - uttara 134
  - yoga 134
- oleation 122-125
- purgation 129-130
  - contraindications 129
  - process 129-130
  - signs of excess bouts 130
- sternutation 130-132
  - contraindications 131
  - process 131-132
- sudation (Swedana) 125-126
  - classification of 125
  - process of 126
  - signs of proper 126
- vomiting 127-129
  - contraindications 127
  - process of 127-128
  - signs of proper 128
  - care after 128-129

Patient, qualities of 15
Physician, attributes of 14-15
Prabhava 54
Prana, types of
- Apana 21, 28
- Prana 20-21, 28
- Samana 21, 28
- Udana 21, 28
- Vyana 21-22, 28

Pregnant lady
- dos and don'ts for 81-82

R

Rasa (taste)
 characteristics of 52-53
 qualities of 27, 54
 signs of diminution of 39
 sources of 52
 treatment of diminution of 40

S

Sama bile 36
Sama mucus 36
 treatment of 36-37
Sama wind
 symptoms of 36
Seasons
 examination of 55-56
 regimens of 56-61
Semen 69, 73, 75
 attributes of 75
 signs of diminution of 39
 treatment of diminution of 40
Sinful acts 64-65
Skin, layers of 84
Soyas, qualities of 24
Strength, examination of 65-66
Sweat
 signs of diminution of 39-40

T

Therapies, kinds of 41
Time, examination of 55
Tissue elements
 functions of 72
 types of 72
Treatment
 four limbs of 14
Tridosa theory 19-46

U

Urine
 signs of diminution of 39
 treatment of 41

V

Vipaka, definition of 54

W

Water, qualities of 22
Wind (Vata)
 qualities of 28-29, 30
 pains caused by aggravation of 37-38
 signs of diminution of 38
 treatment of 40